SKIN CANCER and other DERMATOLOGICAL DISEASES

Prevention & Treatment

2013 Report

A Special Report published by the editors of
Healthy Years
in conjunction with
The David Geffen School of Medicine at UCLA
Division of Dermatology

Skin Cancer and other Dermatological Diseases: Prevention & Treatment

Consulting Editor: Lorraine Young, MD, Clinical Professor, Co-Chief, Clinical Services, David Geffen School of Medicine at UCLA

Author: Jim Brown, PhD
Group Directors, Belvoir Media Group: Diane Muhlfeld, Jay Roland
Creative Director, Belvoir Media Group: Judi Crouse
Production: Mary Francis McGavic
Associate Editor, Belvoir Media Group: Jim Black
Illustrations: Marty Bee

Publisher, Belvoir Media Group: Timothy H. Cole

ISBN: 1-879620-91-X

To order additional copies of this report or for customer service questions, please call 877-300-0253, or write to Health Special Reports, 800 Connecticut Avenue, Norwalk, CT 06854-1631.

This publication is intended to provide readers with accurate and timely medical news and information. It is not intended to give personal medical advice, which should be obtained directly from a physician. We regret that we cannot respond to individual inquiries about personal health matters.

Express written permission is required to reproduce, in any manner, the contents of this publication, either in full or in part. For more information, write to Permissions, Belvoir Media Group, LLC, 800 Connecticut Avenue, Norwalk, CT 06854-1631.

© 2013 Belvoir Media Group LLC

2013

Report on Skin Cancer and other Dermatological Diseases
Prevention & Treatment

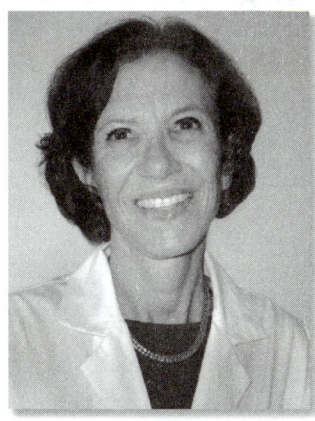

"For the fifth consecutive year, this special report brings encouraging news regarding skin cancer and other skin diseases. The cure rate for all types of skin cancer continues to increase for those who recognize the symptoms and get the appropriate medical care. With early detection, the five-year survival rate is well above 90 percent, and in some cases, as high as 99 percent.

The good news needs to reach more people. In 2012, an American Academy of Dermatology survey found that three of every four Americans do not know that skin cancer is the most common form of all cancer, and only half know how to examine their skin for its signs.

Our hope is that this 2013 edition of *Skin Cancer and Other Dermatological Diseases* will help you become more aware of what you can do to prevent, detect, and treat the most common skin problems.

The mission at the David Geffen School of Medicine at UCLA is to provide quality patient care, to offer evidence-based educational opportunities, and to conduct leading-edge research. This report reflects that mission and will be a valuable resource for you, your family, and your friends.

Thank you for helping us raise the awareness of skin cancer and other skin diseases, and for letting others know that early detection and prompt treatment can lead to a longer, healthier life."

— Lorraine Young, MD, Clinical Professor
Co-Chief, Dermatology Clinical Services
David Geffen School of Medicine at UCLA

HIGHLIGHTS

- Eye color may be an indicator of risk for certain skin diseases. (Page 10, Box 1-2)

- FDA requires sunscreen manufacturers to use simple language on labels. (Page 22, Box 2-6)

- Sunless tanning products may reduce exposure to UV radiation. (Page 23, Box 2-7)

- Indoor tanning rates increase in young women. (Page 24, Box 2-8)

- Half of Americans don't know how to examine their skin for signs of skin cancer. (Page 28, Box 3-1)

- Melanoma rates continue to rise among young adults. (Page 32, Box 3-2)

- Previous cancer elevates risk of melanoma. (Page 33, Box 3-3)

- New melanoma drug may double survival rates. (Page 36, Box 3-6)

- Patients' own tumor-fighting cells promising in resisting melanoma. (Page 36, Box 3-7)

- Experimental drug shrinks secondary tumors in the brain. (Page 36, Box 3-8)

- Melanoma may be triggered by immune system. (Page 37, Box 3-9)

- Progress in developing melanoma vaccine to resist from within. (Page 37, Box 3-10)

- Vitamin A supplements associated with lower melanoma risk. (Page 37, Box 3-11)

- Mohs surgery most cost effective treatment for skin cancer. (Page 41, Box 3-13)

- Picato Gel effective treatment for actinic keratosis. (Page 43, Box 3-14)

- Mixed outcomes for new psoriasis drugs. (Page 51, Box 4-4)

- Shingles vaccine safe and has few side effects. (Page 54, Box 4-5)

Skin Cancer/Dermatological Diseases—2013
A Preview

Chapter 1, More than Skin Deep, describes how the skin protects internal organs, informs the brain, and regulates body temperature. It also highlights an increasing awareness of each person's genetic makeup and its effect on skin health.

Chapter 2, Healthy Skin, presents a consumer-oriented approach to improving skin health. It includes information that can be used in making decisions—from nutrition, sun-safe apparel, and lifestyle choices, to treatment following radiation—that put you in control of your skin's health rather than waiting for something bad to happen.

Chapter 3, Skin Cancer, includes the results of 12 new studies related to the three kinds of skin cancer and a precursor that affect a million new patients every year. The precursor, actinic keratosis, is a particular concern for older adults.

Chapter 4, Other Conditions, is organized into small, easy-to-read segments that serve as a guide for recognizing, treating, and preventing 19 skin conditions all of us have had or might have in the future. This chapter also helps you identify precancerous conditions before they become malignant.

Chapter 5, Getting Help, tells you how to conduct a self-exam, when to seek the help of a dermatologist, and what to expect when you schedule an appointment.

The Appendices include an expanded glossary of 58 terms that you might see in print or hear about regarding skin disease and a list of institutions and organizations where you can get more information.

TABLE OF CONTENTS

Skin Cancer and other Dermatological Diseases—2013 Report

HIGHLIGHTS 4

Chapter 1: More than skin deep 8
    Outer layer—epidermis 8
    Middle layer—dermis 8
    Deepest layer—subcutaneous (subcutis) 9
    Beyond protection 9
    Constant state of change 10
    The gene factor 10

Chapter 2: Healthy skin 12
    Nutrition for healthy skin 13
    Skin-specific vitamins and minerals 13
    Trigger foods 16
    Clothes that protect 17
    Sunglasses that filter 18
    Time of day matters 19
    Smoking ages skin 19
    Sunscreens that help protect 20
    Protection for older adults 23
    Tanning lotions and sprays 23
    Indoor tanning 24
    Radiation treatment 26

Chapter 3: Skin cancer 28
    Basal cell carcinoma 28
    Squamous cell carcinoma 30
    Melanoma 32
    Treatment options for all types of skin cancer 38
    Prevention 41
    Actinic keratosis 42

Health Special Report
PO Box 8545
Big Sandy, TX 75755-8545

Packing Slip/Invoice

Invoice Date: 3/13/13

Amount Due: $28.90

Qty	Item #	Description
1	SR8513	Skin Cancer 2013 Edition

#160103348456#
HSR01600000
JUDY PEHRSON
1181 SPRING GROVE AVE
LANCASTER PA 17603-4936

23
S001/001

Health Special Report
PO Box 8545
Big Sandy, TX 75755-8545

HSR16010334845016000000028907

Please detach this portion and mail today!

16010334845

HSR 16 0 16010334845

Dear Judy Pehrson,

Thank you for your order. This shipment contains:

Qty	Item #	Description
1	SR8513	Skin Cancer 2013 Edition

Please take a moment to examine the attached Packing slip / Invoice to make sure that your name and address are listed correctly. You may mark any corrections on the slip and we'll make the change when you return it to us using the enclosed envelope.

We hope you enjoy reading the enclosed material and appreciate your business.

0328605320

Chapter 4: Other conditions 44
    Aging skin 44
    Age- and illness-related skin care 47
    Psoriasis 49
    Psoriatic arthritis 52
    Shingles 53
    Diabetes-related skin conditions 54
    Boils 57
    Cysts 58
    Dermatitis 59
    Calluses and corns 61
    Skin tags (acrochordon) 62
    Seborrheic keratosis 62
    Rosacea 63
    Sunburn 65
    Moles (nevi) 68
    Hives 69
    Lupus 71
    Warts 72
    Other infections 73
    For more information 74

Chapter 5: Getting help 75
    Self-exam instructions 75
    Seeing a doctor 76
    What to take on the first visit 77
    The exam 77
    Organizations and institutions 77

APPENDIX I: GLOSSARY 78
APPENDIX II: RESOURCES & Contact information 80

1 MORE THAN SKIN DEEP

Skin consists of three layers, and each has its makeup and a specific purpose. Each layer is susceptible to damage caused by neglect, disease, injuries, and the effects of aging. You can take specific steps to maintain the health of all three layers of skin and to avoid, or at least delay, some potentially unhealthy conditions.

Outer layer—epidermis

> **WHAT YOU SHOULD KNOW ABOUT ...**
>
> **Your skin**
> - Skin continues to grow after other tissues, organs, and structures begin to deteriorate with age.
> - Each square half-inch of skin contains 15 sebaceous glands and 100 sweat glands.
> - Most skin cancers appear after the age of 50, but damage caused by the sun begins at an early age.
> - Skin renews itself approximately every four weeks.
> - The average adult uses at least seven different skin care products every day.

The thin, tough outer layer of skin is the epidermis (see Box 1-1). Although only 1/100 of an inch thick, it has three sub-layers. The first is the horny layer, which is continually shedding dead cells. A protein called keratin, produced by those dead cells, protects the skin against harmful outside substances. The second sub-layer of the epidermis contains keratinocytes, or squamous cells, which help protect internal organs, muscles, nerves, and blood vessels. The basal layer is the inner part of the epidermis. Here, basal cells continually divide, forming new keratinocytes and replacing the old ones that are shed from the skin's surface. The process of continuous cell re-newal and shedding takes about a month.

The epidermis also contains cells called melanocytes, which produce the pigment melanin and are largely responsible for the color of skin. Melanin has the more important job of filtering ultraviolet rays (radiation) from sunlight. Damage from the sun causes many problems, the most dangerous of which is skin cancer.

Langerhans' cells, found in the epidermis, are part of the body's immune system. These cells detect and defend the body against foreign elements, but they can also be a factor in the development of skin allergies.

Middle layer—dermis

The thick middle layer of skin is the dermis, which consists of collagen, elastin, and fibrillin that make the skin strong and flexible. It contains blood vessels, lymph vessels, hair follicles, sebaceous glands, and sweat glands, as well as sensory receptors. Some areas of the skin contain more nerve endings than others. The fingertips and toes, for example, are more sensitive to touch than other parts of the body. Skin contains nerves that allow for both pleasant and painful sensations.

Sweat glands produce sweat in hot or stressful situations. When the sweat evaporates, the skin is cooled.

Sebaceous glands secrete sebum in hair follicles. Sebum is an oily substance that protects the skin and keeps it soft and moist.

Blood vessels of the dermis provide necessary skin nutrients and help regulate body temperature. Heat makes them expand to release body heat, and they respond to cold temperatures by constricting and retaining body heat.

Deepest layer—subcutaneous (subcutis)

The deepest layer of skin is called the subcutis, or subcutaneous layer. It holds fat and collagen cells, conserves body heat, holds reserve fuel, and acts as a shock absorber to protect organs from injury.

Beyond protection

The most visible function of our skin is protection against heat, cold, light, infection, chemicals, and injury. But the skin also stores water and fat, and it interacts with sunlight to ensure the production of vitamin D. (See the Nutrition section in Chapter 2.) The amount of water as a component of skin varies with the layer. The outer layer consists of approximately 80 percent water—other layers, between 10 and 30 percent.

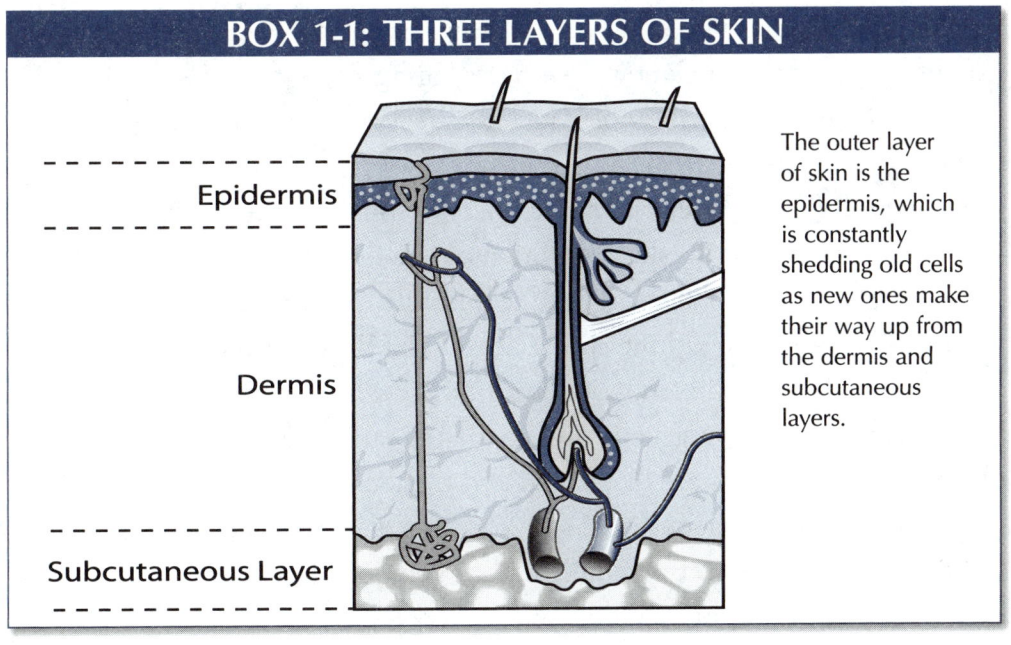

BOX 1-1: THREE LAYERS OF SKIN

The outer layer of skin is the epidermis, which is constantly shedding old cells as new ones make their way up from the dermis and subcutaneous layers.

> **NEW FINDING**
>
> **Box 1-2: Eye color may be an indicator of risk for certain skin diseases**
>
> University of Colorado School of Medicine research suggests that eye color may indicate a higher or lower risk for certain serious skin conditions. A study of approximately 3,000 people revealed that people with blue eyes are less likely to have vitiligo and that people with brown eyes may be less likely to have melanoma. The research team also identified 13 genes that predispose individuals to vitiligo, which is an autoimmune skin disease in which pigment loss results in irregular white patches of skin and hair. People with vitiligo are also at higher risk for other autoimmune diseases such as type 1 diabetes, rheumatoid arthritis, lupus, and thyroid disease. That new finding may lead to greater awareness of the association between genes and other autoimmune diseases.
>
> (*Nature Genetics,* published online May 6, 2012)

All of these functions require a tough, formidable organ, and the skin is our body's largest, weighing six or seven pounds and covering, on average, an area of 21 square feet. It is thickest where it needs to be—on the bottoms of our feet and the palms of our hands. It has extra protection (nails) on the tops of our fingers and toes, and contains hair follicles for more protection and, coincidentally, for appearance.

Scientists once thought each type of cell in the skin had its own stem cell, a type of cell that can produce replacement cells. Now there is evidence that a single type of stem cell, unscientifically called "the mother of all skin cells," is capable of producing all skin cells. This origin of skin cells appears to live in hair follicles.

Constant state of change

Whatever state your skin is in today, change is inevitable—sometimes good, sometimes bad. Every day it sheds old cells and produces new ones. At middle age and beyond, the skin starts to wrinkle, becomes drier, develops "age" or "liver" spots, and may even produce growths. While some of these changes are harmless, others are not and will require medical attention. The important message to remember is that many age-related skin conditions are preventable if you take action early enough and treatable once they develop.

The gene factor

One of the most prevalent trends in skin research is the discovery of how our genes affect not only the nature and appearance of skin, but how our genetic makeup can make us more or less susceptible to skin diseases and conditions. Rosacea, melanoma, shingles, aging skin, psoriasis, psoriatic arthritis, lupus, hives, and moles have a direct genetic component, and there may be others.

Even a physical characteristic like eye color may be an indicator of greater or lesser risks for certain skin conditions. A study conducted at the University of Colorado showed that people with blue eyes are less likely to have vitiligo (an autoimmune skin disease) and those with brown eyes are less likely to have melanoma (see Box 1-2).

Skin cancer has been genetically mapped. That development could change the way these diseases are diagnosed and treated.

Genetics are not a factor in all skin diseases. It is possible to develop any condition mentioned in this report even if you don't have a family history that might make you more vulnerable.

Even though we might have genetic predispositions to some skin diseases and built-in resistance to others, we do not have to be held captive by our genes; nor do they give us a free pass in skin care. Knowing who we are in terms of skin makeup and genetics gives us the advantage of doing something about it—lifestyle choices that involve the foods we eat, how much we weigh, exposure to sunlight, and the environment in which we choose to spend our time. ■

2 HEALTHY SKIN

The American Academy of Dermatology and other organizations offer practical suggestions for protecting aging skin. Below are 10 skin care guidelines for people of any age, with an emphasis on those 40, 50, 60, and beyond.

1. Check your skin daily for dry, red, or irritated skin that might lead to an infection.
2. Stay well hydrated. Fluids will help to keep your skin moist and healthy.
3. Don't smoke. Smoking causes wrinkles and premature aging. Tobacco use narrows the small blood vessels that supply oxygen and nutrients to the outer layers of the skin. Smoking can damage elastin and collagen, which make the skin strong and flexible.
4. Shave carefully. Moisten your skin first (don't shave dry skin), and rinse your skin with warm water after shaving. The idea is not to irritate the skin in a way that could lead to an infection. This is especially important for older adults, whose skin may be thin, dry, or sensitive.
5. Wear cotton underwear that allows air to circulate around the body to keep it comfortably dry.
6. Tell your family physician or dermatologist if you have or suspect a skin problem. After age 40, get a skin examination once a year.
7. Avoid unnecessary exposure to sunlight, and don't use tanning beds. Protection from ultraviolet rays may be the most important way to take care of your skin.
8. Use broad-spectrum sunscreens that have a sun protection factor (SPF) of at least 30. Wear clothing that protects your skin from the sun, and if possible, avoid exposure between 10 a.m. and 4 p.m., when rays are most damaging.
9. Keep your skin clean, but don't overdo it. Washing your hands too often can cause contact dermatitis. Use a mild soap, wash gently, rinse the soap off, and dry your body completely. Check places where water can hide, such as under the arms, between the legs, and between the toes.
10. Use a moisturizing cream or lotion to prevent dry skin after a bath or shower. Your doctor can recommend a commercial product. Some soaps and sunscreens also contain moisturizers.

Nutrition for healthy skin

WHAT YOU SHOULD KNOW ABOUT...

Nutrition and your skin

➤ Older adults need less food to maintain the same weight, but the need for vitamins and minerals to keep the skin healthy stays the same or increases.

➤ Vitamins A, B complex, and C have direct effects on the health of the skin.

➤ Vitamin D deficiency is common among older adults and often goes undiagnosed.

➤ Foods can trigger or aggravate skin conditions such as psoriasis, eczema, and rosacea.

➤ Red beans, wild blueberries, and kidney beans are three excellent sources of anti-oxidants, which protect cells against sun, pollution, wind, temperature, metabo-lism, and the presence of excess oxygen.

From a nutritional standpoint, the best thing you can do for your skin is to eat a well-balanced diet. Most people, however, have only a vague notion of what a well-balanced diet really means. The definition has changed during the past few years, especially if you are in the 50-and-older age group. For example, older adults need less food to maintain the same weight, but the need for vitamins and minerals may stay the same or increase.

Tufts University food scientists developed recommendations to help people age 50 and older eat a healthful diet. Box 2-1 is based on the food pyramid and shows the food group, sources, and recommended number of daily servings.

Skin-specific vitamins and minerals

Several vitamins and antioxidants have a direct or indirect effect on skin health. The antioxidant properties of vitamins appear to help in the prevention and treatment of sun-related skin aging. Nutritional programs could play a role in the "inside out" prevention of skin cancer, meaning that certain foods contain properties that protect against the damage caused by ultraviolet-A radiation. Among the substances that fall into that category are antioxidant vitamins, minerals, and phytochemicals, in addition to polyunsaturated fatty acids. The following is a discussion of those nutrients, as well as examples of sources and their recommended dietary allowances (RDA).

BOX 2-1: DAILY FOOD RECOMMENDATIONS FOR ADULTS 50 AND OLDER

FOOD GROUP	DAILY SERVINGS	SOURCES
Low/non-fat dairy products	3 or more	low or non-fat milk, yogurt, cheese
Meat, fish, poultry, legumes	2 or more	dried beans, fish, skinless poultry, lean meat, eggs
Vegetables	3 or more	romaine lettuce, squash, sweet potatoes, carrots, vegetable juice, spinach
Fruits	2 or more	peaches, bananas, berries, melons, apricots, raisins, orange juice
Grains and cereals	6 or more	raisin bran, oatmeal, whole wheat bread, enriched pasta or rice
Water/liquids	8 glasses	water, tea, coffee, reduced-sodium soup, non-fat milk

Vitamin A

Vitamin A affects the health of epithelial tissue, the lining of the connectors (throat and sinuses) that open to the outside of the body. It also acts as an antioxidant, to offset processes that would lead to wrinkles, and to resist infection. Vitamin A is vital for the growth and repair of cells, tissues, and the skin itself, and it may help relieve allergy symptoms that could manifest on the surface of the skin. Vitamin A helps the skin and mucous membrane (the moist linings of the body's orifices and internal parts) function as a barrier to bacteria and viruses. If an older person does not get enough vitamin A, he or she could develop dry skin, itchy skin, and loss of skin elasticity.
- Sources: eggs, milk, sweet potatoes, fruits, vegetables
- RDA: 900 micrograms (mcg) for men; 700 mcg for women

Vitamin B complex

Vitamin B complex includes riboflavin, niacin, vitamins B-6 and B-12, and biotin. Biotin is a substance needed to grow skin, nail, and hair cells. Niacin helps the skin retain moisture, but too much can cause the skin to flush (as it does when heart patients take niacin supplements) and, in more severe cases, liver damage. A vitamin B complex deficiency could result in dry, flaky, or sensitive skin.
- Sources: whole grains, whole-grain cereals, rice, oatmeal, eggs, fish, dairy products
- RDA: Vitamin B-6—1.3 milligrams (mg) for adults age 19-50, 1.7 mg for men 51 and older, and 1.5 mg for women 51 and older; Vitamin B-12—2.4 mcg; Riboflavin—1.3 mg for men, 1.1 mg for women; Niacin—16 mg for men, 14 mg for women; Biotin—30-100 mcg

Vitamin B3 (niacin) may have potential in treating photoaging, but more trials are needed before making a definitive statement regarding its specific role.

Vitamin C

Vitamin C helps the body produce collagen and elastin, both of which are needed for healthy, firm skin. It protects the skin against infections and facilitates the healing process. When you have a vitamin C deficiency, wounds may not heal as rapidly as they should. The National Institutes of Health (NIH) recognizes vitamin C as an antioxidant that blocks damage caused by free radicals (unstable molecules produced during normal metabolism, when food is turned into energy). The accumulation of free radicals is partially responsible for the aging process. Vitamin C may reverse the negative effects of UV radiation, but there are few clinically controlled studies to confirm this theory.

- ■ Sources: citrus fruits and fruit juices, broccoli, berries, dark green leafy vegetables
- ■ RDA: 90 mg for men, 75 mg for women

Vitamin D

Skin plays a vital role in the natural production of vitamin D. When ultraviolet rays from sunlight strike the skin, they trigger the synthesis of vitamin D, which is essential for many functions of the body, including bone health. Vitamin D is also contained in foods and supplements, but long-term calcium and vitamin D supplementation does not appear to reduce the rate of non-melanoma skin cancer. Vitamin D deficiency, however, is very common among older adults and often goes unrecognized by physicians.

Exposure to sunlight is perhaps the most important source of vitamin D, which makes for a controversial issue among health care professionals. Too much sun exposure is known to cause skin cancer. Too little sunlight inhibits the body's production of vitamin D. The benefits of limited sun exposure appear to outweigh the risks of developing skin cancer, but not all dermatologists are convinced.

The American Academy of Dermatology's position statement on vitamin D makes it clear that exposure to sunlight is not recommended as a means of obtaining vitamin D. Instead, vitamin D should be obtained from a healthy diet that includes foods naturally rich in vitamin D, foods and beverages fortified with vitamin D, and/or other vitamin D supplements.

Sensible sun exposure—five to 10 minutes on the arms, legs and face, two or three times per week—and increased dietary and supplemental intakes are reasonable options for getting sufficient vitamin D. For those with limited sun exposure, it is especially important to include good sources of vitamin D in their diets and to use supplements as directed by their physician.

- ■ Sources: sunlight, dairy products, fatty fish (such as tuna or mackerel), fortified cereals, eggs, beef, liver
- ■ RDA: 600 international units (IUs) for adults up to age 70; 800 IUs for adults age 71 and older

Vitamin E

Vitamin E has antioxidant properties, fights damage caused by free radicals, and has the potential for slowing the aging process. We have learned that UV exposure significantly decreases levels of cutaneous (skin) vitamin E, and vitamin C should be included in any formulation containing vitamin E because of its role in maintaining vitamin E levels.

- Sources: green leafy vegetables, broccoli, almonds
- RDA: 15 mg

Zinc

Zinc is needed for general skin health, repairing skin damage, and providing firmness, elasticity, and strength to the skin. When the body is zinc-deficient, its resistance to infection is compromised.

- Sources: meat, fish, oysters, egg yolk, milk, whole grains, liver
- RDA: 11 mg for adult men; 8 mg for adult women

Antioxidants

Antioxidants are a recurring theme in nutrition and skin care (see vitamins A, C, and E). According to the National Cancer Institute, antioxidants are substances that protect cells from the damage caused by free radicals. Free radicals may play a part in cancer, heart disease, stroke, and other diseases of aging, and they are detrimental to skin health. Box 2-2 lists the top 20 food sources of antioxidants, in order of total antioxidant capacity per serving.

Selenium

Although selenium is an essential trace mineral that is good for health, selenium supplements apparently have no role in the prevention of skin cancer. Earlier observational studies suggested that selenium supplementation might have been associated with a lower risk. The *Cochrane Database of Systematic Reviews* found no evidence that taking selenium supplements lessens the risk of non-melanoma skin cancer.

Trigger foods

A well-balanced diet is important for good skin care. However, some foods can worsen certain skin conditions. For example, rosacea is triggered in some people by spicy foods, alcohol, soy sauce, dairy products, hot

BOX 2-2: FOOD SOURCES OF ANTIOXIDANTS*

RANK	FOOD	SERVING SIZE
ITEMS	SERVING SIZE	½ cup
1	Small red beans (dried)	½ cup
2	Wild blueberries	1 cup
3	Red kidney beans (dried)	½ cup
4	Pinto beans	½ cup
5	Blueberries	1 cup
6	Cranberries	1 cup
7	Artichoke (hearts)	1 cup
8	Blackberries	1 cup
9	Prunes	½ cup
10	Raspberries	1 cup
11	Strawberries	1 cup
12	Red Delicious apples	1
13	Granny Smith apples	1
14	Pecans	1 ounce
15	Sweet cherries	1 cup
16	Black plums	1
17	Russet potatoes (cooked)	1
18	Black beans (dried)	½ cup
19	Plums	1
20	Gala apples	1

* *Journal of Agricultural and Food Chemistry*, June 2004.

chocolate, hot cider, tea, and coffee. Milk, eggs, peanuts, soy, wheat, fish, chocolate, and tomatoes might worsen eczema symptoms. Psoriasis can be triggered by alcohol, and alcohol may diminish the effectiveness of psoriasis treatments. Food-related skin problems are an individual matter, and something that causes an episode in one person may not do the same in another. Read more about rosacea, eczema, and psoriasis in Chapter 4.

Clothes that protect

> **WHAT YOU SHOULD KNOW ABOUT...**
>
> **Sun-protective clothing**
>
> ➤ The higher the ultraviolet protection factor (UPF) in clothing, the better.
> ➤ If you can see light through a piece of clothing, it does not offer adequate protection.
> ➤ Dark-colored clothes provide more protection than light-colored garments.
> ➤ Wet clothes can lose up to 50 percent of their UPF capacity.
> ➤ For clothes that provide protection, look for the Skin Cancer Foundation's *Seal of Recommendation* on the label.

Clothes can protect skin against ultraviolet (UV) rays, but the weave, weight, fiber, color, and amount of skin covered determine the amount of protection they provide. The Skin Cancer Foundation and other organizations use the ultraviolet protection factor (UPF) system to indicate how much UV radiation a fabric absorbs (see Box 2-3).

A fabric with a UPF of 50 allows only 1/50th (about two percent) of the sun's UV rays to pass through, and will significantly reduce radiation exposure. The higher the UPF, the better. Only clothes with a UPF of 15 to 50+ can carry a label that says "sun-protective." These clothes usually have a UPF of 50+. But like regular fabrics, sun-protective clothes can lose their effectiveness if they are pulled too tight, stretched, or washed and worn often.

If you want to buy or use clothing or other products that effectively block the sun's rays, look for the Skin Cancer Foundation's *Seal of Recommendation* on the label. Download a complete list of products that have earned the *Seal of Recommendation* at http://www.skincancer.org/seal/.

Light-colored, lightweight, and loosely woven fabrics provide very little protection against the sun. White T-shirts provide an average UPF of only seven, while a long-sleeved, dark, denim shirt offers a UPF of about 1,700—almost a complete sun block. To informally check a fabric for its sun-blocking ability, hold it up to a light. If you can see through it, UV radiation can penetrate it and do its damage.

Dark-colored fabrics are more effective at blocking sunlight than light-colored ones. Thicker fabrics also offer more protection—for example, velvet in black, blue, or dark green gets a UPF rating of 50. Fabrics such

BOX 2-3
Ultraviolet protection factor (UPF) ratings

VALUE	AMOUNT OF PROTECTION
50	Maximum protection
40-49	Excellent protection
25-39	Very good protection
15-24	Good protection

as unbleached cotton contain special pigments that absorb UV rays, while certain polyesters and even thin, satiny silk can be very protective because they reflect radiation. The problem is that these kinds of fabrics may not be fashionable or practical in situations where the potential for UV damage is high (beaches, water, mountains). If you can't wear long pants and a long-sleeved shirt or blouse, boost your protection by staying in the shade as much as possible and by applying a sunscreen with an SPF of at least 30.

What you do while wearing a particular fabric can make a difference. If the fabric gets stretched, it loses some of its protective ability because it becomes thinner and more permeable. Wet fabrics can lose up to 50 percent of their UPF. In Florida, parents often put a white T-shirt on their children to protect them from the sun while swimming, but that wet T-shirt has a UPF of only three.

Consider buying and wearing fabrics that have been treated with chemical UV absorbers, called colorless dyes. They prevent both main types of ultraviolet rays (UVA and UVB) from penetrating the fabric and reaching the skin. Some companies make sun-protective clothing that has been treated with a chemical sun block during the manufacturing process.

An additive called Sun Guard (available from drugstores and online at www.sunguardsunprotection.com) can be added to laundry detergent to increase the UPF rating of clothing without changing the texture or color. It is effective for up to 20 washings.

A hat can shield your skin from UV rays if it provides shade for everything that will be exposed to the sun. Wear a hat with a brim wide enough to protect your face, ears, and back of your neck. A baseball cap is better than nothing, but not much better. Darker hats provide more protection than lighter caps, and tightly woven caps, such as those made of canvas, protect better than loosely woven caps and hats. Don't wear straw hats with holes that allow sunlight to get through.

Sunglasses that filter

Wear sunglasses that block both UVA and UVB rays. The majority of sunglasses sold in the United States meet this standard, according to the U.S. Centers for Disease Control and Prevention. Wraparound sunglasses are best because they block sun-light from getting in at the sides of the glasses. Here are some other suggestions from The Glaucoma Foundation:

- Always choose sunglasses labeled as blocking 99-100 percent of UV rays. Some manufacturers' labels say "UV absorption up to 400nm," which means the same thing as 100 percent UV absorption.

- Consider "fitover" sunglasses that can be worn over your regular prescription glasses.
- Use sunglasses that screen out 75-90 percent of visible light. Try the glasses on in front of a mirror. If you can see your eyes easily through the lenses, they probably are too light.
- Look for a uniform tint, not darker in one area than in another.

Time of day matters

The sun's rays are strongest and capable of the most damage from 10 a.m. until 4 p.m. Reduce your risk of skin damage by staying inside during that time period and by seeking shade or using an umbrella. Even staying in the shade does not guarantee protection. UV rays can reflect off almost any surface, including sand, snow, concrete, and asphalt, and get to your skin. Don't take chances—protect your skin when you are outside, regardless of available shade.

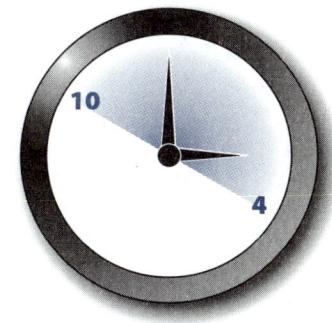

Avoid exposure to the sun between 10 a.m. and 4 p.m.

Smoking ages skin

WHAT YOU SHOULD KNOW ABOUT...

Smoking and aging skin

- Smoking accelerates the skin aging process by 10-20 years.
- Signs of aging skin in smokers begin at age 20.
- Smoking leads to a breakdown of collagen needed for skin health.
- Smoking blocks the absorption of vitamin C.
- Some skin damage caused by smoking is reversible.

More than a decade of research has established a very strong connection between smoking tobacco and accelerated skin aging. The American Academy of Dermatology reports that cigarette smoking causes biochemical changes that speed up the aging process in the skin and other organs. A person who smokes at least 10 cigarettes a day for 10 years is more likely than a nonsmoker to develop wrinkled, leathery skin. Even when the wrinkling is not normally visible, the process can be seen under a microscope in smokers as young as age 20. Long-term smokers may also develop a yellowish or ashy tint and dullish appearance to their complexion.

Smoking is associated with a higher degree of aging on areas of the skin not normally exposed to sunlight, such as the inside of the upper arm. The total number of packs of cigarettes smoked per day and the number of years a person smokes have been linked to the amount of skin damage a person experiences. Among those age 45 or older, the degree of skin aging is significantly higher in smokers than nonsmokers. It is even more pronounced among smokers in the 65-and-older age group.

Previous research has documented the effects of smoking, exposure to the sun, a history of outdoor activities, and the lack of sunscreen use with the older appearance of skin. Even though some people have the same genetic makeup, sun damage can be compounded by smoking, being overweight, and failure to use sunscreen.

Smoking may add between 10 and 20 years to the natural aging of a person's skin. The damage is caused by the following factors:

- Restricted blood flow through the capillaries that supply oxygen and nutrients to the skin.
- Increased production of an enzyme that breaks down the supply of collagen to the structure of the skin.
- Reduced stores of vitamin A, which protects against skin damage.
- Blocked absorption of vitamin C, which is needed for skin protection and health.
- Increased deeply wrinkled skin around the eyes and mouth—both symptoms of "smoker's face."

Some of the skin damage caused by smoking cannot be reversed, but those who stop smoking, eat a healthful diet, protect themselves from the sun, and take regular care of their skin can get back a few of the 10-20 years lost due to smoking.

Sunscreens that help protect

> **WHAT YOU SHOULD KNOW ABOUT...**
>
> **Sunscreens**
>
> ➤ Sun protection factor (SPF) refers to a sunscreen's ability to screen or block the sun's rays.
>
> ➤ Dermatologists recommend an SPF sunscreen of 15 (preferably 30) year-round.
>
> ➤ UVB rays are more responsible for sunburn, while UVA rays penetrate more deeply and are more responsible for underlying skin damage.
>
> ➤ Broad-spectrum sunscreens protect against UVA and UVB radiation.
>
> ➤ No sunscreen can block 100 percent of dangerous UV rays.

The best way to avoid skin damage caused by the sun is to stay inside, especially during peak daylight hours. Less exposure to the sun is better than any kind of protection against its rays. The second best strategy is to wear clothing that protects the skin, and the third most effective measure is to apply sunscreen.

There are three kinds of ultraviolet rays emitted by the sun—UVA, UVB, and UVC—but for now, only A and B reach the Earth's surface. As the ozone layer that surrounds the Earth thins or develops holes, UVC rays may begin contributing to sunburn and premature aging of the skin. UVA rays penetrate the skin more deeply than UVB rays and are associated with making wrinkling, sagging, and other skin problems worse than they should be (see Box 2-4). They also seem to compound the cancer-causing effects of UVB rays, which are primarily responsible for sunburn. UVA and UVB rays are dangerous in their own ways, and your skin needs protection against both.

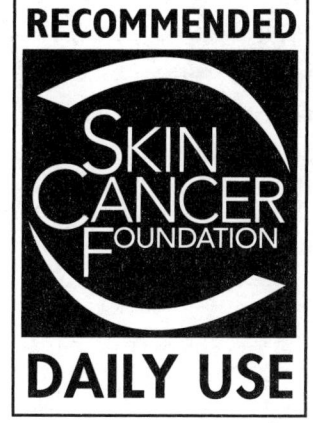
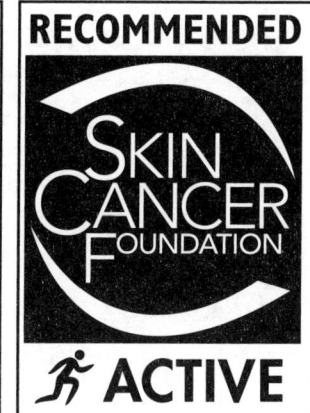

Sunscreens are all based on a sun protection factor (SPF) system, which is a measurement of the sunscreen's ability to prevent UVB from damaging the skin. The higher the number, the better the protection, but it is not an absolute scale. A sunscreen with a 15 rating means that you can be exposed to the sun's rays without damage 15 times longer than you could without a sunscreen. A sunscreen with a 15 SPF filters approximately 93 percent of UVB rays, a 30 SPF filters about 97 percent, and a 50 SPF blocks 99 percent.

The Skin Cancer Foundation has implemented new standards for sunscreens in its Seal of Recommendation program. These new standards include rigorous UVA protection requirements, and sunscreens will be divided into two categories based on their intended use. "Daily Use" products are intended to protect from incidental sun exposure that occurs over short periods of time. "Active" products should protect against extended sun exposure.

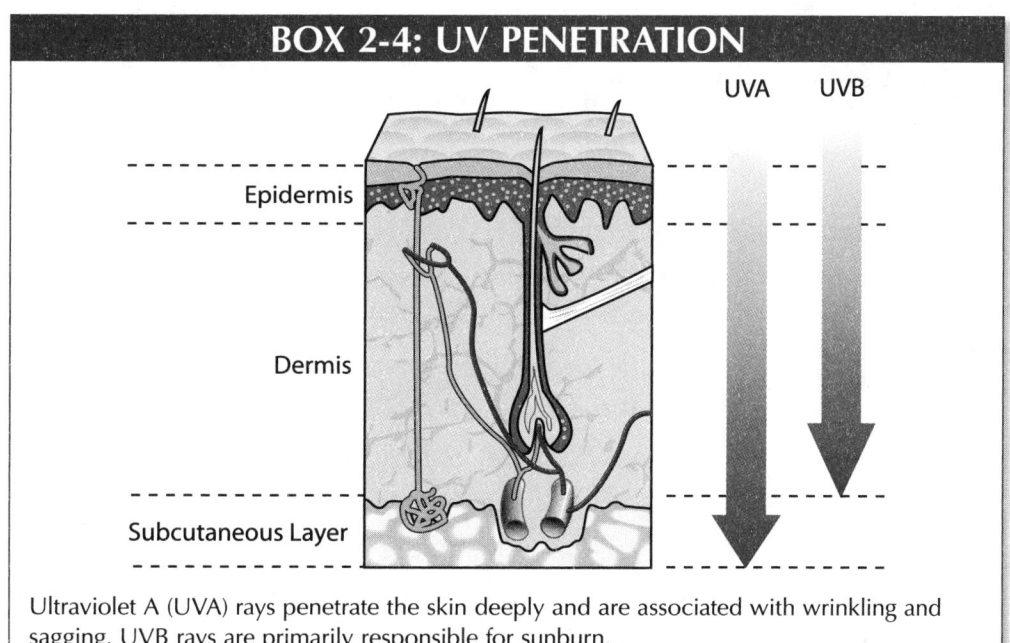

BOX 2-4: UV PENETRATION

Ultraviolet A (UVA) rays penetrate the skin deeply and are associated with wrinkling and sagging. UVB rays are primarily responsible for sunburn.

BOX 2-5: EFFECTIVENESS OF SUNSCREEN INGREDIENTS*

SUNSCREEN INGREDIENT	TYPE	PROTECTION	
		UVA	UVB
p-Aminobenzoic acid (PABA)	Chemical	Minimal	Extensive
Avobenzone	Chemical	Extensive	Limited
Cinoxate	Chemical	Limited	Extensive
Dioxybenzone	Chemical	Considerable	Extensive
Ecamsule	Chemical	Extensive	Limited
Homosalate	Chemical	Minimal	Extensive
Methyl anthranilate	Chemical	Considerable	Extensive
Octocrylene	Chemical	Limited	Extensive
Octyl methoxycinnamate	Chemical	Limited	Extensive
Octyl salicylate	Chemical	Limited	Extensive
Oxybenzone	Chemical	Considerable	Extensive
Padimate O	Chemical	Minimal	Extensive
Phenylbenzimidazole	Chemical	Minimal	Extensive
Sulisobenzone	Chemical	Considerable	Extensive
Titanium dioxide	Physical	Considerable	Extensive
Trolamine salicylate	Chemical	Minimal	Extensive
Zinc oxide	Physical	Extensive	Extensive

* Adapted from "The Burning Facts," U.S. Environmental Protection Agency, 2006.

NEW REGULATIONS

Box 2-6: FDA requires sunscreen manufacturers to use simpler language on labels

As of December 17, 2012, sunscreen manufacturers were to be required by the Food and Drug Administration to include easier-to-understand labels on sunscreen products. Among the new regulations:

Sunscreens cannot be labeled "sunblock."

To be labeled "broad" spectrum," sunscreens must provide equal protection against UVA and UVB radiation.

The words "waterproof" and "sweatproof" cannot be used, only how long after application they are effective.

The term "instant protection" or words to the effect of "protects skin for more than two hours" cannot be used unless the FDA approves them for the sunscreen in question.

Labels must be clear about how much sun protection factor (SPF) the product provides.

(Food and Drug Administration, December 2012)

Physical sunscreens form a protective film that reflects UV light before it can penetrate the skin. They contain substances such as zinc oxide and titanium dioxide, both of which protect against UVA and UVB rays. Chemical sunscreens absorb UV rays instead of reflecting them. They contain avobenzone or oxybenzone. Parsol 1789 is the trade name for a sunscreen that contains avobenzone.

Box 2-5 lists ingredients found in various sunscreens, the type of protection they offer, and effectiveness of protection against UVA and UVB rays. Notice that zinc oxide is the only ingredient that provides extensive protection against both UVA and UVB radiation.

Use a broad-spectrum sunscreen that contains more than one chemical and can protect against both kinds of rays, as well as doing a better job of protecting your skin against photo (light) damage and rashes caused by sun exposure.

Don't forget to protect your lips with a lip sun block of at least 30 SPF. Shiny lip balms and glosses may attract ultraviolet rays and increase the risk of skin cancer. Less than 25 percent of Americans use some form of lip protection.

No sunscreen can block 100 percent of dangerous rays, and none of them are perfect. They offer protection for two hours at best and less time in conditions of high humidity, sweating, drying or rubbing your skin with a towel, and any contact with water, including swimming. Sunscreen guidelines always include a suggestion to re-apply the product at least every two hours. Sunscreen can't be waterproof, but it can be water-resistant.

As of December 17, 2012, the Food and Drug Administration instituted new regulations designed to make sunscreen manufacturers use simpler language on labels. See Box 2-6 for a list of terms that are prohibited or that must be clarified.

Guidelines

In spite of compelling evidence regarding the benefits of using a sunscreen, most people do not use these products properly. Less than 30 percent of the population uses pre-applied sunscreen, and 41 percent of those who do use it don't apply it until they have already been in the sun long enough to cause damage. Follow these guidelines for sunscreen use provided by the Skin Cancer Foundation, the Mayo Clinic, and other institutions:

- Apply sunscreen 15-30 minutes before going out into the sun.
- Use broad-spectrum, water-resistant sunscreens.
- Generously apply a sunscreen with at least a 15 SPF (preferably 30).
- Reapply every two hours, even on cloudy days, and after swimming or sweating.
- Seek shade when appropriate.
- Avoid exposure to the sun's rays between 10 a.m. and 4 p.m.
- Don't use color of skin (redness) to indicate skin damage. Sunburned skin may take 24 hours to turn red.
- The FDA is in the process of developing new requirements for UVA coverage in sunscreens and for sunscreen labeling changes.

Protection for older adults

Aging skin declines in its ability to repair damage produced by sun exposure. Also, cumulative light damage results in thin, damaged skin that worsens with additional exposure. Older adults have skin that is less effective at sweating and cooling, so they should wear lightweight, tightly woven clothing that covers exposed skin surfaces. They should also plan outdoor activities when the sun is not directly over-head and the air is cooler.

Even driving habits can increase the risk of sun damage. Skin cancers develop predominantly on the left side of drivers—the side more likely to be exposed to the sun while driving.

Tanning lotions and sprays

Tanning lotions, creams, and sprays are safe; tanning beds are not. A study conducted at Emory University found that the frequent use of sunless tanning products was associated with less exposure to UV radiation from other tanning methods (see Box 2-7). Lotions contain a substance that interacts with

---

NEW FINDING

Box 2-7: Sunless tanning products can reduce exposure to ultraviolet radiation (UV)

At Emory University, researchers found that frequent use of sunless tanning products (STP) is associated with less exposure to UV radiation from other tanning methods, such as exposure to sunlight and using tanning beds. More than 400 women were surveyed regarding their tanning habits and attitudes. Of those who used tanning products, 36.8 percent reported having decreased their intentional sun exposure because of STP use. Among those who also used tanning beds, 38 percent said they had reduced their tanning bed use. More than 90 percent of the women believe that tanned skin is more attractive than non-tanned skin, a perception that is likely to lead to frequent tanning habits, regardless of the method used.

(*Archives of Dermatology,* April 2012)

proteins in the skin to produce a tan-like color, but the SPF factor is negligible. You'll still need a sunscreen with at least an SPF of 15 (preferably 30). Tanning beds present a health risk. Ultraviolet light, wherever it comes from, can cause skin cancer and wrinkling.

Indoor tanning

> **WHAT YOU SHOULD KNOW ABOUT...**
>
> **Indoor tanning**
>
> ➤ Indoor ultraviolet tanners are 74 percent more likely to develop melanoma than those who have never tanned indoors.
>
> ➤ People who use tanning beds are 2.5 times more likely to develop squamous cell carcinoma and 1.5 times more likely to develop basal cell carcinoma.
>
> ➤ Ten minutes in a sunbed matches the cancer-causing effects of 10 minutes in the Mediterranean summer sun.
>
> ➤ Almost 30 people tan indoors in the U.S. every year.
>
> ➤ Eighteen percent of Americans over the age of 50 use indoor tanning devices.
>
> (Adapted from Skin Cancer Foundation)

In spite of negative publicity and warnings from private and government health organizations, about one million Americans use tanning beds every day, according to the Health Physics Society. Almost one-third of white women between the ages of 18 and 21 use indoor tanning devices at least once a year (see Box 2-8), and of women who do report indoor tanning an average of 28 times during a 12-month period.

Use of tanning beds is not limited to younger adults. Approximately eight percent of adults 65 and older use tanning beds, as do 10 percent of those in the 50 to 64 age group and 14 percent of adults 40 to 49 years old.

Some people still don't understand the danger, others choose to ignore the risks of tanning in favor of "looking good," and still others simply can't help themselves. The American Academy of Dermatology reported in one study that 72 percent of 7,000 survey respondents agreed that people with tans look more attractive and 66 percent felt that tanned skin looks healthier even though it is not. An *Archives of Dermatology* study found some people can actually become addicted to tanning, and that those people are more likely to show signs of anxiety and use of certain drugs.

NEW FINDING

Box 2-8: Indoor tanning rates increase in young white women

Thirty-two percent of white women between the ages of 18 and 21 use indoor tanning devices at least once during a 12-month period. Women in that group reported indoor tanning an average of 28 times during the one-year period. The numbers are "astounding" according to an American Cancer Society official, especially in light of the fact that experts have been warning that exposure to ultraviolet radiation from the sun and indoor tanning equipment dramatically increases the risk of skin cancer. Overall, 5.6 percent of adults reported indoor tanning during the past 12 months. A previous study showed that people who use tanning beds are 74 percent more likely to develop melanoma.

(*Morbidity and Mortality Weekly Report,* May 11, 2012)

Excessive sunlight has been associated with skin cancer for more than 100 years, and tanning beds emit the same types of ultraviolet rays as the sun. The quantity and quality of research continues to increase. A decade ago the U.S. Department of Health and Human Services stated that tanning beds and sunlamps "are known to be a human carcinogen."

People who have used indoor tanning beds have an increased risk of developing melanoma, and the risk is even greater among those whose first use was before age 35. Parents and guardians tend to pass their indoor tanning habits onto their children.

Exposure to UV rays from tanning beds increases the risk of melanoma. Sunlamps that emit ultraviolet rays may also pose a risk for skin cancer. A modest association exists between sunlamp use and melanoma, but the risk increases with frequency and duration of use.

The University of Iowa provides a summary of the evidence regarding sunlamps and tanning beds. The report says that people who used tanning beds before age 35 have a risk of melanoma eight times greater than those who have never used them. In addition, those who use tanning beds are:

- 2.5 times more likely to develop squamous cell carcinoma.
- 1.5 times more likely to develop basal cell carcinoma.
- More likely to develop basal cell and squamous cell carcinoma the younger they were when they began using tanning devices.
- Have a 74 percent higher rate of melanoma than those who have never used the devices.

The U.S. Food and Drug Administration (FDA) says the effects of tanning beds and sunlamps can be as dangerous as tanning outdoors. Some devices emit only UVA rays, while others produce both UVA and UVB rays. The FDA says there is limited evidence to support claims that artificial tanning via lamps and beds is less dangerous because the intensity and duration of tanning are controlled. In fact, sunlamps may be more dangerous than the sun because they can be used with equal intensity year-round, which is unlikely for the sun because of winter weather and cloud cover.

The American Academy of Dermatology points out that most sunlamps and tanning beds emit only UVA radiation. However, UVA rays penetrate the skin more deeply, and they have been associated with the development of melanoma. Both UVA and UVB have also been linked to damage of the immune system and premature skin aging.

International Agency for Research on Cancer, a working committee of the World Health Organization, includes tanning beds and lamps on the list of cancer-causing devices and substances that emit dangerous levels of ultraviolet radiation.

The Health Physics Society warns that tanning booths are especially dangerous for the eyes. Ultraviolet radiation levels to the eye could be more than 100 times greater in a tanning booth than outside in the sun. Corneal burns, cataracts, and retinal damage can occur.

FDA guidelines for using tanning beds

Some people will begin using or continue using sunlamps and tanning beds in spite of overwhelming evidence of their potential harms. They should adhere to the following guidelines:

- Wear goggles that fit snugly and are not cracked.
- Use short exposure times and build up a tan over time.
- Do not use maximum exposure time with first use.
- Follow manufacturer-recommended exposure time for your skin type.
- Stick to your time limit.
- After developing a tan, use a tanning bed no more than once a week.

Radiation treatment

Radiation produced by the sun's rays (UVA and UVB) is mentioned or discussed throughout this report. Radiation produced during routine X-ray procedures, mammographies, computed tomography (CT) scans, and fluoroscopy accumulates throughout a lifetime, but is not associated with permanent skin damage.

Radiation therapy is used to treat 50-60 percent of cancer patients, and it can have a temporary effect on the skin. In fact, skin reactions and fatigue are the two most common side effects. The skin reactions depend on the area of the body, as well as the amount and type of radiation. Whatever the type, radiation therapy destroys the ability of cancer cells to reproduce, and the body eventually gets rid of them.

Side effects of radiation therapy include red, dry, irritated, or peeling skin. In some patients, the skin develops a dark or bronze appearance, and other patients have a reaction in which the skin is moist and sore—usually in areas where the skin folds. These reactions are more noticeable among patients who are undergoing radiation and chemotherapy at the same time, but they can also occur in those who are receiving radiation treatment only.

Skin reactions to radiation become noticeable within two or three weeks after treatment has begun, and they start to subside about three weeks after the last treatment. Your radiologist will give you specific instructions about how to care for your skin during and after a series of radiation treatments.

Guidelines

The following is a composite list of ways to care for your skin while undergoing radiation treatment. The list is long, but following the instructions will make you more comfortable and your treatment more effective.

- Keep the radiated area dry and free from irritation. Cornstarch patted on with a powder puff can help keep the skin dry.
- Wash the area with mild soaps (Dove, Ivory, Neutrogena, Basis, Castile, Aveeno Oatmeal Soap), but be careful not to wash off skin markings.
- Do not scratch, rub, or irritate the area.
- Do not use any product that contains alcohol.
- Do not apply cosmetics, shaving lotions or creams, perfumes, or deodorants to the treated area.
- Wear loose-fitting, soft, lightweight, cotton clothing. Avoid wool, corduroy, or garments that have been starched.
- Women who are being treated for breast cancer should avoid wearing bras.
- Do not expose the area to extreme heat or cold—no heating pads, hot water bottles, or ice applications.
- Keep baths and showers as short as possible.
- Use an electric razor if you have to shave the area.
- Stay out of direct sunlight, and use a sunscreen with an SPF of at least 15 (preferably 30) when you have to be in the sun.
- Do not use adhesive tape or Band-Aids on the treated area.
- Check with your radiologist if you have questions or skin problems, especially if you experience blistering, swelling, or tenderness.
- Follow these skin care measures for two to three weeks after radiation therapy has been completed, and avoid direct exposure to the sun for at least a year.

(Sources: The Ohio State University, Cleveland Clinic, American Society of Radiologic Technologists, U.S. Food and Drug Administration)

3 SKIN CANCER

> **WHAT YOU SHOULD KNOW ABOUT...**
>
> **Skin cancer**
>
> ➤ 3.5 million new cases of skin cancer are diagnosed each year.
> ➤ One in five Americans will develop skin cancer.
> ➤ 75 percent of skin cancer deaths are from melanoma.
> ➤ The incidence of melanoma has been rising for 30 years.
> ➤ Unprotected sun exposure is the most preventable risk factor for skin cancer.
>
> *(from the American Academy of Dermatology)*

Skin cancer is responsible for a third of all cancers in the United States, and nearly half of all Americans who live to age 65 will develop skin cancer at least once. The incidence of non-melanoma skin cancer cases is higher than previously thought, according to the American Academy of Dermatology. The total number now exceeds three and a half million, and that does not include middle-aged and younger adults.

Awareness of the prevalence of skin cancer and knowledge of how to perform self-exams is regrettably low. Three of four Americans do not know that skin cancer is the most common type of cancer in the U.S., and little more than half know how to examine their bodies for signs of the disease (see Box 3-1).

There are three kinds of skin cancer—basal cell carcinoma, squamous cell carcinoma, and melanoma. Susceptibility, warning signs, diagnosis, treatment, and prevention are discussed in the following sections for each type, and a more detailed description of all treatments appears near the end of this chapter.

Basal cell carcinoma

> **WHAT YOU SHOULD KNOW ABOUT...**
>
> **Basal cell carcinoma**
>
> ➤ Basal cell carcinoma is the most common form of skin cancer.
> ➤ There are one million new cases every year.
> ➤ Overexposure to the sun is responsible for 90 percent of all skin cancers, including basal cell carcinoma.
> ➤ Basal cell carcinoma is treatable and curable when diagnosed early.
> ➤ Fair-skinned individuals who burn easily are most susceptible.

Basal cell carcinomas (BCC) are slow-growing, painless malignant tumors that develop in the epidermis, the top layer of skin. They almost never spread, but if left untreated, they can affect surrounding areas and even move into bone tissue.

BCC is the most common form of skin cancer. It is classified as a non-melanoma form of the condition, and it accounts for about 75 percent of all skin cancer cases. In 2012, approximately one million new cases of BCC will have been reported. The cure rate is 85-99 percent.

NEW FINDING

Box 3-1: Half of Americans don't know how to examine their skin for signs of skin cancer

The results of a survey conducted by the American Academy of Dermatology showed that 74 percent of Americans did not know that skin cancer is the most common form of cancer in the U.S. In addition, only half (53 percent) knew how to examine their skins for signs of cancer, and 30 percent were either unsure or did not know that skin cancer can be easily treated when detected early. Respondents who knew how to examine their skin were more than twice as likely to have shown suspicious moles or spots to a medical professional as those who did not know.

(American Academy of Dermatology Survey, May 2012)

Who is susceptible?

People who spend a lot of time outdoors, those who are fair-skinned, and those who live in areas of the country where there is more sunlight per day (Arizona, Texas, and Florida) are at a higher risk for BCC and other forms of skin cancer. Others in the high-risk group are people with blue or green eyes, blond or red hair, and those who have been over-exposed to X-rays and other forms of radiation. At one time, BCC was more common among people over age 40, but it is increasingly being diagnosed in younger adults.

The number one cause of basal cell carcinoma is exposure to sunlight (the sun can be blamed for 90 percent of all skin cancers, including BCC). The areas of the body most likely to be affected are the face, ears, neck, scalp, and back.

Warning signs

The warning signs of basal cell carcinoma are an open sore that bleeds, a sore that doesn't heal, oozing or crusting areas in a sore, scar-like sores in an area that has not been injured, irregularly-shaped blood vessels in or around the spot, or a sore that has a depressed area in the middle. Other ways to describe a potential cancer are a reddish patch of skin, a shiny bump, and a pink growth.

There are seven subtypes of basal cell carcinoma, but the most common is a nodular BCC. It usually has a smooth, round, waxy area that could be yellow or gray, and it varies in size from one centimeter to a few millimeters. The slightest irritation to the lesion can cause bleeding. Large nodular BCCs are easy to diagnose, but small ones may resemble warts, moles, psoriasis, or other noncancerous skin conditions.

Diagnosis

A skin biopsy can confirm whether or not an area of the skin is cancerous, and if so, which type of skin cancer exists. Biopsies are conducted in the office of a dermatologist, who uses a topical analgesic to prepare the site. Tell your doctor if you are allergic to lidocaine or other types of local anesthesia. He or she will perform a biopsy—either a shave or a punch—which involves using a sharp instrument to cut and remove the appropriate skin tissue. For a suspected melanoma, the entire lesion may be removed. The sample is then sent to a pathologist, who examines the skin sample under a microscope and determines its status. If it is a melanoma, additional surgery is usually necessary.

Treatment

The treatment for basal cell carcinoma depends on its size, location, and depth. Simply scraping the affected area off or cutting it away are common ways of treating this condition.

However, when the cancer reaches an advanced state, surgery is not always an option. In 2012, though, the FDA approved vismodegib (Erivedge) to treat adult patients with basal cell carcinoma. The drug is intended for use in patients with locally advanced basal cell cancer who are not candidates for surgery or radiation, and for patients whose cancer has spread to other parts of the body (metastatic). Visomodegib is the first drug of its kind to help advanced basal cell carcinoma patients who have few treatment options. The drug can help shrink a tumor by targeting something called the "hedgehog signaling pathway," a group of molecules in a cell that help control certain cell functions. In adults, the hedgehog signaling pathway can lead to basal cell carcinoma. Vismodegib helps shut down the troublesome pathway.

A study published in the June 7, 2012, online edition of the *New England Journal of Medicine* also demonstrated that vismodegib (Erivedge) can dramatically shrink basal cell cancers, as well as prevent the formation of new ones in patients with a rare genetic conditions called basal cell nevus syndrome. The drug is not recommended for the treatment of basal cell carcinoma in the general population.

Prevention

The recurring theme for prevention of skin cancer is to limit exposure to the sun's rays. Avoid being in the sun altogether, when possible, during midday hours, and protect yourself against its rays at other times by using sunscreen with an SPF of at least 15 (preferably 30), or wearing pants, long skirts, long-sleeved shirts, and wide-brimmed hats.

Squamous cell carcinoma

> **WHAT YOU SHOULD KNOW ABOUT...**
>
> **Squamous cell carcinoma**
> - It is the second most common form of skin cancer.
> - Middle-aged and older adults are most susceptible.
> - 250,000 new cases are reported every year.
> - Most cases are caused by overexposure to sunlight.
> - 95 percent of cases can be cured if treated early.

Squamous cell carcinoma (SCC) is the second most common form of skin cancer, and about 250,000 new cases are diagnosed in the U.S. each year. With early identification and treatment, the five-year survival rate is 95-98 percent. If untreated, SCC can spread to other organs and tissues, which results in approximately 2,500 deaths per year. Once it has spread, the five-year survival rate drops to below 50 percent.

Who is susceptible?

The people most likely to get SCC are middle-aged and older adults. Other risk factors are fair complexions, frequent exposure to the sun, a history of working in the sun, early childhood over-exposure to the sun, getting artificial tans in tanning beds, and living in an area of high-intensity sunlight. Women living in the southern part of the United States have almost twice the risk of developing SCC as those residing in the North. However, geographic location does not appear to be related to incidence of melanoma, but location on the body does. The thicker a skin cancer tumor, the more likely it is to spread, and squamous cell carcinomas on or near the ears are four times more likely to spread than those elsewhere on the body.

You are also at greater risk if you have light-colored hair and blue, green, or gray eyes. Exposure to radiation, arsenic, and other chemicals increases the risk. Finally, you are more susceptible to SCC if you have had any previous type of skin cancer, or if you have a weakened immune system as a result of disease or chemotherapy.

Hispanics, Asians, and African-Americans are much less likely than Caucasians to develop SCC, but more than two-thirds of skin cancers that affect darker-skinned people are SCCs.

Warning signs

The cancer appears as a rough, scaly bump that grows, and the surface of the lesion may also have a flat, reddish patch. It usually occurs on the face, ears, neck, hands, or arms, but can develop elsewhere.

The warning signs of SCC include a sore that doesn't heal, a change in a mole or wart, and a rough, scaly, reddish bump that appears to be growing.

Diagnosis

The condition is diagnosed by a biopsy conducted in a dermatologist's office. The tissue is sent to a pathologist to determine whether or not it is cancerous.

Treatment

If the entire lesion was removed as part of the biopsy, the primary treatment is over. If further treatment is necessary, surgery, laser surgery,

NEW FINDING

Box 3-2: Melanoma rates continue to rise among young adults

Research at Mayo Clinic revealed that the incidence of melanoma increased by eight times among young American women and by four times among young men from 1970 through 2009. The researchers studied first-time diagnoses of melanoma in patients between the ages of 18 and 39. Although the rate of melanoma has increased, the number of people who are dying from skin cancer has decreased. Early detection and treatment are likely to be the reasons for improved survival rates.

(*Mayo Clinic Proceedings*, April 2012)

---

cryosurgery, radiation therapy, and electrodesiccation and curettage (scraping and cauterizing the tumor) are options.

Anyone who has had SCC or any other type of skin cancer should have frequent follow-up appointments, and every adult should have an annual skin examination by a physician or dermatologist. Remember that a person who has had one skin tumor has a 40 percent risk of developing a new lesion within two years, and all tumors are not evident to the patient.

Prevention

Avoid sun exposure, and protect your skin by wearing clothes that shade the arms, legs, face, neck, and ears.

Melanoma

WHAT YOU SHOULD KNOW ABOUT...

Melanoma

➤ Melanoma is the most serious form of skin cancer and resulted in new 75,000 cases in 2012.

➤ One in 70 Americans will develop the condition at some point.

➤ With early detection, the survival rate is 99 percent.

➤ Fair-skinned, sun-sensitive individuals are at highest risk.

➤ Overexposure to the sun is the most preventable cause of melanoma.

When melanoma is detected before it reaches deeper than the outer layers of the skin, the five-year survival rate is 99 percent. When detected later, the survival rate drops to below 50 percent, and in some cases below 20 percent.

More than 100,000 new cases of melanoma are diagnosed each year, and more than 8,000 people die from the disease. Melanoma accounts for 75 percent of all skin cancer deaths, and about one in 70 Americans can expect to develop the condition at some point. Despite efforts at improving prevention, the incidence of invasive melanoma is rising by four to six percent annually in the U.S. The increase is particularly high among young adults between the ages of 18 and 39. In April, 2012, *Mayo Clinic Proceedings* reported that the incidence of melanoma increased by eight times among young American women and by four times among men over a 40-year period (see Box 3-2).

The risk of melanoma is nine times higher in people with a history of the skin malignancy as it is in the general population. People who survive melanoma not only have a greater risk of a second melanoma, but also of 12 other types of cancer.

Conversely, people who have survived breast cancer, Kaposi sarcoma, lymphoma, or other skin cancers have an increased risk for cutaneous melanoma, according to a study published in *Archives of Dermatology* (see Box 3-3).

Who is susceptible?

Anyone can develop melanoma, but the profile is much clearer for this type of skin cancer than for others: Fair-skinned, sun-sensitive people are at higher risk, especially redheads, blonds, and people with blue or green eyes. The more moles, large moles, and unusual moles, the more likely a person is to eventually have a melanoma. The risk of melanoma also may be inherited. You are more likely to have the condition if either of your parents, children, siblings, cousins, aunts, or uncles has had a melanoma. Your chances increase if you've had a previous melanoma, a basal cell carcinoma, or a squamous cell carcinoma.

Here are five risk factors associated with developing melanoma:

- History of a previous melanoma
- Age over 50
- No regular contact with a dermatologist
- A mole that is changing
- Male gender

A history of sunburns, red or blond hair, freckles on the upper back, family history of melanoma, and outdoor summer jobs early in life have shown to be reliable predictors of future melanoma.

Dark hair and complexion of skin, once thought to be associated with a degree of protection, appears to be a reliable predictor. Gene mutations appear to be more important than either the hair or skin color factors. A change in the BRAF gene may be the first step in a series of genetic changes that eventually leads to melanoma.

Researchers have found that location on the body may be an indicator of fatal melanomas. Melanomas on the scalp and neck are more likely to be fatal than those at other sites. However, atypical moles are not limited to any area of the body. They can occur anywhere.

Surprisingly, people with a family history of melanoma are twice as likely to develop Parkinson's disease than those with no history of the condition. There might be genetic characteristics common to both diseases. Researchers have also recently discovered that people with Parkinson's disease appear to have an increased risk of melanoma and prostate cancer.

Biomarkers

Identifying melanoma biomarkers has been the focus of research on at least three fronts. Scientists at Yale identified a group of plasma biomarkers

---

NEW FINDING

Box 3-3: Previous cancer elevates risk of melanoma

People who have survived breast cancer, Kaposi sarcoma, lymphoma, or other skin cancers have an increased risk for cutaneous melanoma (CM). CM is the fifth most commonly diagnosed cancer in the U.S. among men and the seventh most common among women. Researchers analyzed the medical records of more than 70,000 patients who had developed CM as a first primary cancer and more than 6,000 patients who were diagnosed with CM after surviving a previous cancer. Those with a previous cancer diagnosis were at a significantly higher risk. The results suggest the need for continued skin monitoring among melanoma and selected other cancer survivors.

(*Archives of Dermatology*, December 2011)

BOX 3-4

Differences between a normal mole and melanoma

Normal mole

- Circular shape; both halves match
- Smooth, regular borders
- Single color
- Diameter smaller than a pencil eraser

Melanoma

- One side or half of the mole does not match the other
- Irregular, ragged borders
- Color varies throughout the area
- Diameter larger than a pencil eraser

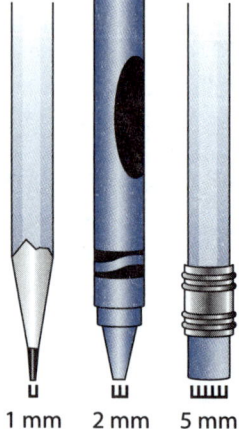

that could eventually predict the risk of melanoma spreading to other parts of the body. At the University of North Carolina, a team confirmed that a type of testing called DNA methylation distinguishes malignant and non-malignant moles. Researchers at Boston University identified a molecule that plays an important role in the metastasis process. Targeting the molecule could inhibit cancer cell growth.

Warning signs

Melanoma is characterized by uncontrolled growth of cells (melanocytes) that produce the pigment melanin, one of the body's coloring agents. Most melanomas have a black or blue-black color, and they tend to look abnormal, if not ugly. The American Academy of Dermatology, the American Cancer Society, and the Skin Cancer Foundation widely publicize the following A, B, C, D, E method of identifying potential melanomas:

- **A—Asymmetry.** The shape of one half of the lesion does not match the other half.
- **B—Border.** The edges are ragged, notched, blurred, or otherwise irregular.
- **C—Color.** The color of the area is not uniform and could include shades of brown, black, and tan, with streaks of red, white, or blue.
- **D—Diameter.** Melanomas are usually greater than six millimeters (about a quarter-inch) when diagnosed, but they can be smaller.
- **E—Evolving, as in the illustration below.** The growth is changing in size, shape, color, or thickness, or it's starting to itch, bleed, and form a crust.

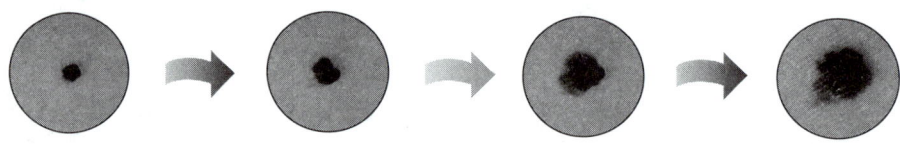

If you see these warning signs or if you notice a change in a mole, contact a dermatologist as soon as possible (Box 3-4). Go to www.melanoma-monday.org/ for more information from the AAD about detecting melanoma, including a downloadable Body Mole Map.

The deeper a melanoma has penetrated, the more deadly it becomes. If it reaches beyond lymph nodes in the immediate area, the five-year survival rate is only 18 percent.

Diagnosis

A variety of methods is used to diagnose melanomas, including a medical history, biopsies, and imaging tests. Melanomas are classified and treated according to stages of development. Stages are determined by 1) how deeply the tumor has penetrated the skin, 2) ulceration (a break on the surface of the tumor), 3) involvement of lymph nodes, and 4) metastasis (spread to distant organs). Five-year survival rates depend on the stage, and stages are subdivided by the letters A, B, and C, with C more severe than A (see Box 3-5).

A type of melanoma most likely to affect adults ages 50 to 80 is lentigo maligna melanoma (LMM). In its early stage, LMM appears as a flat, dark patch. It tends to develop on skin that has been exposed to the sun over a long period of time, and it may be mistaken for a large age spot or freckle.

Treatment

Early-stage melanomas can easily be removed by simple procedures at a dermatologist's office. In some cases, the entire area in question can be excised (cut out) during a biopsy, requiring no further treatment. Melanomas that have spread beyond the surface of the skin are more difficult to treat with surgery, but this treatment approach may address the symptoms for several years. In Mohs micrographic surgery—used for delicate areas, such as the nose, lips and ears—the surgeon uses a microscope to examine the tissue and excises the growth layer by layer until only healthy tissue remains.

Chemotherapy

Chemotherapy, in pill or intravenous form, destroys cancer cells for several months, but the treatment does not have a good record of curing melanomas. New drugs such as riluzole, vemurafenib, and ipilimumab are being tested, and older ones may still relieve symptoms.

BOX 3-5: MELANOMA STAGES, TREATMENT OPTIONS, AND SURVIVAL RATE

STAGE	TREATMENT	SURVIVAL RATE
0	surgery (excision); creams	89-100%
1	surgery to remove the melanoma and surrounding skin	>90%
2	surgery; lymph node biopsy and excision, if necessary	45-79%
3	excision of primary tumor and lymph nodes; interferon to lower risk of recurrence; possible radiation, chemotherapy	30-69%
4	surgery, chemotherapy, immunotherapy, biochemotherapy	7-19%

Source: American Cancer Society

Research presented at a meeting of the American Society of Clinical Oncology found that ipilimumab extended survival rates of 25 percent of stage III and IV melanoma patients by two years. The drug may be even more effective if given earlier in the course of the disease and to patients who are less ill. The Food and Drug Administration approved the use of ipilimumab (Yervoy) for advanced melanoma in March 2011, and in June 2011, separate research found that Yervoy combined with another drug increased survival rates over the three-year period. In addition, research showed that the drug vemurafenib (also called PLX4032) resulted in a 74 percent reduction in the progression of melanoma and a 63 percent reduction in the risk of death.

Researchers at Vanderbilt found that a drug called vemurafenib nearly doubled the survival rate of 132 melanoma patients (see Box 3-6).

At the Fred Hutchinson Cancer Research Center, a small study revealed that chemotherapy combined with patients' tumor-resistant T-cells was promising in treating advanced melanoma (see Box 3-7).

And finally, Australian scientists used an experimental drug called dabrafenib treat a gene mutation that causes melanoma and in the process, found that the drug may also shrink secondary tumors in the brains of patients with advanced forms of the disease (see Box 3-8).

Radiation

Radiation can kill cancer cells, including those produced in melanoma, but this treatment is not considered a cure for melanoma. Fatigue is a common side effect of radiation that usually, but not always, subsides after treatment has been completed.

Immunotherapy

Immunotherapy (biological) therapy is an attempt to stimulate a person's immune system to resist tumor cells. The *New England Journal of Medicine* reported that a vaccine for advanced melanoma improved

---

NEW FINDING

Box 3-6: New melanoma drug may double survival rates

Researchers at Vanderbilt and 12 other centers in the U.S. and Australia found that the new drug vemurafenib (Zelboraf) nearly doubles the survival rates of melanoma patients. Of the 132 subjects in the study, half were treated with the novel drug. Survival increased from the average rate of six to 10 months to nearly 16 months for patients whose melanoma had spread beyond the original tumor site. Although previous studies had been conducted with vemurafenib, this was the first to confirm the durability (extended time period) of the response.

(*New England Journal of Medicine,* February 23, 2012)

NEW FINDING

Box 3-7: Patients' own tumor-fighting cells promising in resisting melanoma

A small study conducted at the Fred Hutchinson Cancer Research Center in Seattle found that patients' own tumor-resistant T-cells combined with chemotherapy appears to be a promising approach in treating advanced melanoma. Of the 11 subjects, one experienced long-term, complete remission and in four others, the melanoma temporarily stopped growing. If scientists can develop methods to grow these types of cells in the laboratory, all patients may eventually benefit from T-cell therapy.

(*Proceedings of the National Academy of Sciences,* March 5, 2012)

NEW FINDING

Box 3-8: Experimental melanoma drug shrinks secondary tumors in the brain

An experimental drug called dabrafenib that targets a gene mutation of melanoma may also shrink secondary tumors in the brains of patients with advanced forms of the disease. Secondary tumors are those that have spread from the original site. Most patients with brain metastases die within four months. In this trial, conducted in Australia, the brain tumors shrank in nine of the 10 patients within the first six weeks. All 10 patients survived beyond five months and two survived beyond 12 months. If further trials are successful, dabrafenib may address a large unmet need in patients with metastatic melanoma.

(*The Lancet,* May 18, 2012)

response rate and survival when combined with the immunotherapy drug interleukin-2.

Scientists at Yale and Johns Hopkins found that melanoma could be caused by the immune system turning on itself (see Box 3-9). Among patients with tumors containing the B7-H1 molecule, when the immune system tried to suppress the inflammatory response, growth of their tumors increased. New therapies might be able to block the immune-suppressing ability of the body in this specific case.

Another inside-out approach showed promise at Mayo Clinic and the University of Leeds. Scientists used animal studies to train the immune systems to eradicate skin cancer from within by using a combination of human DNA combined with a virus. "Cancer immunotherapy" may be able to identify a new set of genes to stimulate the immune system to reject cancer (see Box 3-10).

Regardless of the treatment recommended, men and women appear to react differently after being diagnosed and treated for melanoma. Men appear to be less aware of ways to protect against the sun than women, while women may need more counseling to cope with melanoma than men.

Prevention

There are four basic ways to avoid any kind of skin cancer, including melanoma: 1) Avoid unnecessary sun exposure. 2) Use a minimum SPF 30 sunscreen that protects against both UVA and UVB rays. 3) Wear clothes that protect your arms, legs, face, neck, and ears. 4) Conduct a monthly skin self-exam and schedule annual exams performed by a dermatologist.

A study conducted in Washington suggests a diet-related fifth way to lessen the risk of melanoma. Researchers analyzed data on 70,000 people for a five-year period and found that those who took vitamin A supplements had a 40 percent lower risk of developing the disease (see Box 3-11). The authors do not (yet) recommend taking a

---

NEW FINDING

Box 3-9: Melanoma may be triggered by the immune system

Scientists at Yale School of Medicine and Johns Hopkins Medical Institutes found that melanoma might be triggered when the immune system turns on itself. The researchers focused on a specific immune-inhibiting molecule called B7-H1, which is found in melanoma tumors. Among patients with tumors containing the molecule, suppression of the inflammatory response hastened the growth and aggressiveness of their tumors. The team also found that tumor cells use a component of the immune system to turn on B7-H1 and suppress the immune system. The finding makes it possible to develop therapies that block the immune-suppressing ability of the body.

(*Science Translational Medicine,* March 28, 2012)

NEW FINDING

Box 3-10: Progress in developing a melanoma vaccine to resist skin cancer from within

In animal studies, researchers at Mayo Clinic and the University of Leeds (UK) have trained immune systems to eradicate skin cancer from within by using a genetic combination of human DNA and a virus similar to that found in rabies. The approach is called cancer immunotherapy, in which a broad spectrum of genes derived from melanoma cancer cells is delivered directly into tumors. The new technique is expected to identify a new set of genes that encode antigens and stimulate the immune system to reject cancer.

(*Nature Biotechnology,* March 19, 2012)

NEW FINDING

Box 3-11: Vitamin A supplements associated with lower melanoma risk

Vitamin A supplements might lessen the risk of melanoma according to a recent study. The supplement contains retinol, which could be the protective factor. Kaiser Permanente Northern California researchers collected data on approximately 70,000 people for a period of five years and found that those who took vitamin A supplements had a 40 percent less chance of developing melanoma. The study did not, however, prove a cause-and-effect relationship and the authors did not recommend that people start taking vitamin A supplements to prevent melanoma. Diet should remain the number one source of retinol.

(*Journal of Investigative Dermatology,* published online March 1, 2012)

vitamin A supplement specifically to prevent melanoma, but the findings are noteworthy.

An Australian study showed that adults who use a sunscreen during the course of daily activities can drastically reduce their risk of melanoma, but the results do not apply for those who seek intentional exposure to the sun.

Researchers at Penn State University used a compound called ISC-4 that could reduce expansion of melanoma lesions by up to 90 percent. More tests are needed before the substance will be available for clinical use.

Treatment options for all types of skin cancer

The possibility that non-melanoma skin cancer will recur after treatment is less than five percent. A dermatologist or surgeon might choose one or more of the following methods to treat any of the three main types of skin cancer:

Electrodesiccation & curettage

This treatment involves scraping away the cancerous area with a tool called a curette, followed by electrodessication and curettage (ED&C), in which an electrical current is applied to the area through a needle to stop the flow of blood and to get rid of any cancer cells that might have been left behind, especially those around the edges of the wound. Electrodesiccation works best for small, superficial skin cancers such as basal cell carcinoma. A biopsy can determine the extent of skin cancers and whether they might be small enough to treat with electrodesiccation.

Excisional surgery

In excisional surgery, the lesion is surgically removed. Usually performed in a doctor's office under local anesthesia, the procedure has a high cure rate, produces minimal scarring, and can be completed in one session. In more severe cases, this technique requires the removal of nearby healthy tissue. Excision is one of the primary methods of treating melanoma, but in cases where the tumor has spread to other areas of the body, other forms of treatment may be needed.

Cryosurgery

Used to treat basal cell and squamous cell carcinomas, cryosurgery destroys cancer cells by freezing them. The dermatologist sprays the area with liquid nitrogen to freeze it; then the skin is thawed and the process is repeated. The tissue dies and falls off over the next 24 hours. Cryosurgery can be performed in a doctor's office, and generally has a good cure rate. However, it may leave a scar, and it may take several weeks to heal completely.

Chemotherapy

Chemotherapy is the use of oral or intravenous drugs to kill cancer cells. The Food and Drug Administration (FDA) have approved three late-stage melanoma treatments. Dacarbazine is administered intravenously to destroy tumor cells, but its effectiveness is 20 percent at best, and patients survive for an average of only eight months after treatment. Interleukin and interleukin-2 are used during immunotherapy. However, fewer than 20 percent of patients respond to this treatment, and only half of them see a lasting remission of the disease.

Research suggests new ways in which chemotherapy might be effective in treating melanoma. A drug called riluzole appears to slow the growth of highly aggressive melanoma. A combination of two biotherapies—interferon alfa-2b and tremelimumab—might be beneficial for patients with inoperable melanoma.

In addition, promising clinical studies continue on a new drug known as PLX4032, which is administered orally. Studies at the University of Pennsylvania among a small group of patients whose tumors contain a cancer-causing mutation called BRAF have shown both tumor shrinkage and a delay in tumor progression.

Finally, high blood levels of a protein, interleukin-12, appear be an indicator of poor survival rates among patients with advanced melanoma. The finding is evidence that a dys-functional immune system response fuels the growth of tumors.

Radiation

Radiation uses high-energy X-rays and other forms of radiation to kill cancer cells when the cancer has spread to other organs and tissue. It also might be used for tumors that cannot be treated with surgery. In one form, a machine sends radiation to the affected area. In another technique, a needle or catheter places a radioactive substance into or near the cancer.

Laser surgery

Laser therapy, or laser surgery, uses high-intensity light to treat several diseases, including basal cell skin cancer. The beam of light vaporizes the growth. The advantages include minimal bleeding, swelling, or scarring, and little damage is done to surrounding tissues. Laser therapy seems to work best with superficial skin cancers and precancerous growths, to reduce scars following skin cancer surgery, and to treat a variety of non-cancerous skin growths.

Photodynamic therapy

This treatment for precancerous skin lesions uses a combination of laser light and drugs to kill light-sensitive cancer cells. If you choose this option, you'll have to avoid direct sunlight for at least six weeks after the procedure.

Mohs micrographic surgery

Mohs micrographic surgery is a procedure in which each layer of skin is removed and immediately examined (see Box 3-12). The process continues until the skin sample is cancer-free. Mohs surgery is often used for skin cancers that recur, for cancers embedded in scar tissue, and for cancers on the face and other areas where excision or other types of surgeries might not be cosmetically acceptable. The procedure is also preferred when the cancer is extensive and grows very quickly, or when it is difficult to determine the extent of the lesion. Mohs has a very high cure rate for basal cell and squamous cell carcinomas.

Patients who have Mohs surgery to treat basal cell carcinoma have only a one percent chance that the cancer will return. According to the Skin Cancer Foundation, the technique has several major advantages, including preserving more normal tissue, allowing the surgeon to identify and eradicate areas of the tumor that are not normally seen, and providing information that tells the surgeon exactly how far the tumor extends. Also, Mohs surgery does not require general anesthesia, and it is particularly suitable for areas around the eyes, ears, nose, and mouth, where preservation of normal tissue is essential.

Mohs surgery is an outpatient procedure usually performed under local anesthesia or at times with mild sedation. Patients usually return home immediately and have a rapid recovery.

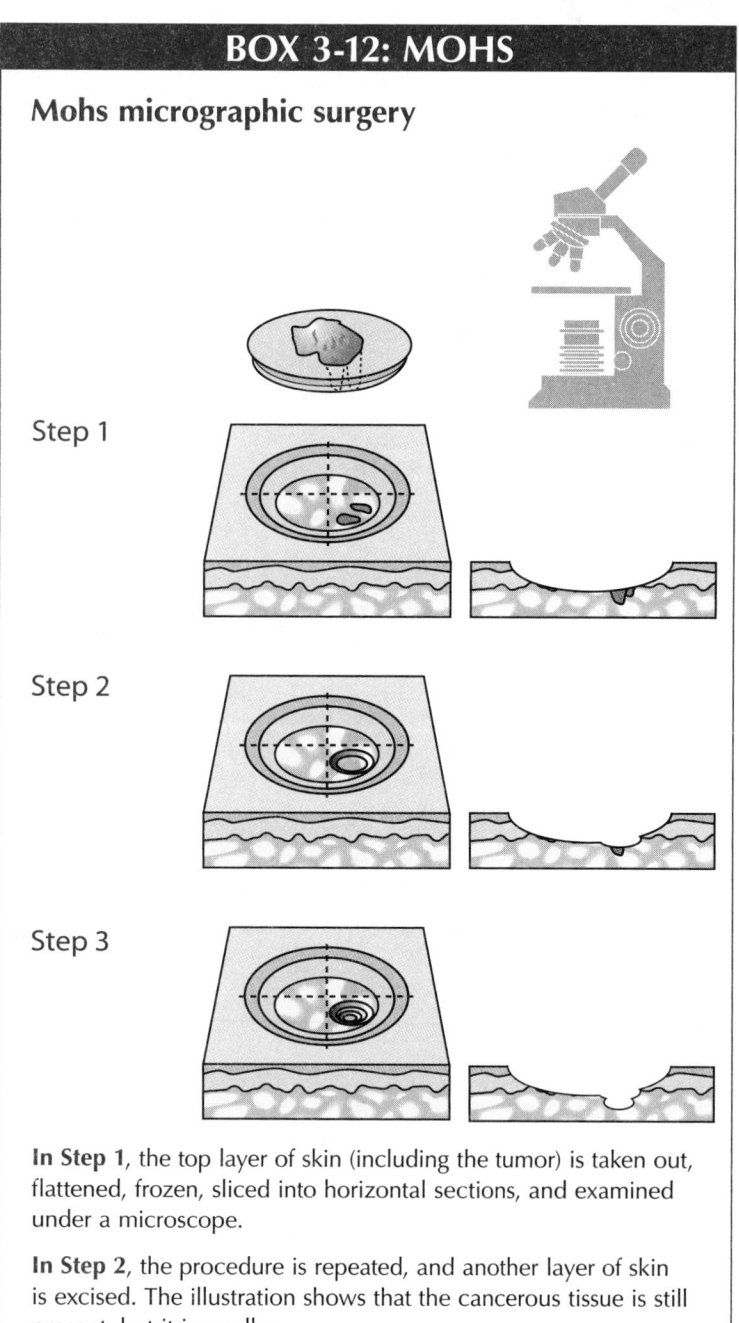

BOX 3-12: MOHS

Mohs micrographic surgery

In Step 1, the top layer of skin (including the tumor) is taken out, flattened, frozen, sliced into horizontal sections, and examined under a microscope.

In Step 2, the procedure is repeated, and another layer of skin is excised. The illustration shows that the cancerous tissue is still present, but it is smaller.

In Step 3, successive layers of skin are removed until the sample tissue is free of the tumor, both vertically and around the edges.

Research conducted at Ohio State and published in the journal *Dermatologic Surgery* showed that Mohs remains the most cost-effective treatment for skin cancer (see Box 3-13).

The disadvantages of Mohs surgery are that the physician has to be specially trained as a surgeon and pathologist, the procedure takes several hours, and some cancers are too large or inaccessible. Cancer that has spread to lymph glands or other tissues is not treatable with Mohs. The success rate in terms of recurrence, according to the *Archives of Dermatology,* is 96.5 percent.

Immunotherapy

Immunotherapy is still being studied. The treatment involves using medications such as interferon and interleukin-2 to stimulate the immune system to fight skin cancer. Other medications, such as imiquimod (Aldara), are applied to the skin and are designed to enhance a person's immune reaction to skin cancer.

Prevention

The ways to reduce your chances of getting any type of cancer are essentially the same. The list of suggestions that follows applies to basal cell carcinoma, squamous cell carcinoma, melanoma, and precancerous skin lesions.

1. Wear long-sleeved shirts and pants, as well as sunglasses and a wide-brimmed hat, to protect your skin from the sun.
2. Use a water-resistant sunscreen with a sun protection factor (SPF) of at least 15 (preferably 30) that protects against both ultraviolet A (UVA) and ultraviolet B (UVB) rays. Don't forget to reapply every two hours and after sweating or swimming. Sunscreens that contain titanium and mexoryl help to block UVA rays.
3. Stay in the shade when possible. The strongest rays of the sun occur between 10 a.m. and 4 p.m. One rule of thumb: If your shadow is shorter than you are, get out of the sun.
4. Be especially cautious when you are near water, snow, or sand. All three reflect the sun's rays, even in the shade, and all three increase your chance of sunburn.
5. Avoid tanning beds. They are an invitation to increase your risk of melanoma.
6. Check your skin at least once a month, and report any changes to your doctor.
7. If you are older than 40, see a dermatologist once a year for a thorough skin examination.

NEW FINDING

Box 3-13: Mohs micrographic surgery most cost-effective treatment for skin cancer

Research at Ohio State and the University of Pittsburgh showed that Mohs micrographic surgery (MMS) represents the most cost effective treatment for skin cancer. The cost of MMS was compared to standard surgical excision (SSE) with permanent margins and SSE with frozen margins. Four hundred and six tumors were included in the study, and the cost comparison confirmed that Mohs is the most cost-effective treatment, regardless of place of service or type of margin control. Adjusted for inflation and including initial examination, biopsy, and five-year follow-up, the cost was $1,376—approximately $250 less expensive than similar procedures 10 years prior to the present study.

(*Dermatologic Surgery,* April 2012)

8. Be aware that some medications—including antibiotics, nonsteroidal anti-inflammatory drugs such as ibuprofen, and some cholesterol, hypertension, and diabetes medications—can make your skin more sensitive to sunlight.

Early-stage melanoma can be cured in almost every case. Later stages of the disease may be treated and sometimes cured, but five-year survival rates drop dramatically. There are arguably more things you can do personally to prevent melanoma than for any other type of cancer.

Actinic keratosis

> **WHAT YOU SHOULD KNOW ABOUT...**
>
> **Actinic keratosis (AK)**
>
> ► The two main causes are exposure to carcinogens (as in the sun's rays) and genetic makeup.
>
> ► Between 40 and 60 percent of squamous cell carcinomas begin as AK.
>
> ► It is most common in fair-skinned persons who have had long-term exposure to the sun.
>
> ► The areas of the body most likely to be affected are the face, scalp, back of the hands, neck, and forearms.
>
> ► The incidence of AK among adults over 40 is between 40 and 60 percent.

There are several kinds of precancerous skin conditions, but the most common is actinic (or solar) keratosis (AK). Lesions from AK are referred to as precancerous because they represent a warning sign and can turn into malignant tumors. Forty to 60 percent of all squamous cell carcinomas begin as AKs, and there is recent evidence that the two are linked genetically. At least 89 unique genes appear in people who have had one or both conditions.

Like many basal cell and squamous cell carcinomas, AKs are likely to be caused by cumulative exposure to the sun's rays. There is also a genetic component to the condition because it occurs most often in sun-sensitive, light-skinned, light- or red-haired individuals with blue or green eyes. Those who live in sunny areas are more susceptible than residents of northern climates.

AKs develop in areas of the skin frequently exposed to the sun, such as the face, scalp, back of the hands, ears, neck, and forearms. They are much easier to diagnosis than basal cell carcinomas, squamous cell carcinomas, and melanomas. In fact, untrained individuals can often recognize them. The affected area is a rough or crusty and dry skin lesion that is limited to a relatively small area—usually between an eighth and a quarter-inch, although some lesions have been as large as an inch in diameter. They may be gray, pink, red, or the same color as the skin, and they may itch or cause a pricking or tender sensation.

Diagnosis may be as simple as a visual inspection by a dermatologist, but a biopsy can be performed to determine if potentially cancerous changes are present.

Treatment

When symptoms of AK are recognized early, the lesions are almost always treatable. Treatment depends on the location of the lesion, its size, and the age, health, and preference of the patient. For example, some people might not prefer a treatment that is very effective but leaves a scar. Fortunately, there are many other treatment options, including cryosurgery, electrodesiccation, photodynamic therapy, laser therapy, and dermabrasion. In dermabrasion, also called surgical skin planing, the dermatologist freezes an area of skin and removes it with a rotary instrument.

Medicated creams (5-fluorouracil is an example) work well on the ears, neck, and face, and are cosmetically acceptable.

Imiquimod cream is an FDA-approved substance that stimulates the immune system by causing cells to produce interferon, which can destroy cancerous and precancerous cells. Studies published in the *Journal of the American Academy of Dermatology* found that imiquimod (Aldara) completely or partially cleared lesions on the face and scalp in 25 and 43 percent of patients, respectively.

A combination gel treatment consisting of hyaluronic acid and a nonsteroidal anti-inflammatory drug called diclofenac is a third topical treatment option.

In March of 2012, Mount Sinai School of Medicine reported in the *New England Journal of Medicine* that Picato Gel (ingenol mebutate) was an effective treatment up to 43 percent of the time among 900 patients in the study. The gel appears to be unique in that it takes a relatively short period of time to clear AK (see Box 3-14).

Chemical peels use an acidic substance applied to the skin that causes the top layers to come off. Those layers are replaced within a week or so by new skin. The only draw-backs are discoloration and irritation.

Prevention

As with skin cancer, AKs might be prevented by staying in the shade instead of unnecessarily exposing the skin to the sun, avoiding direct sunlight between 10 a.m. and 4 p.m., and applying a broad-spectrum sunscreen with an SPF of 15 or greater at least 30 minutes before going out into the sun. Wearing protective clothing and performing regular skin self-examinations are other pre-emptive strikes against skin cancer and precancerous conditions. The rule of thumb for seeing a dermatologist is to schedule an appointment if any area looks suspicious. If something on your skin is growing, assume that it is cancer unless a dermatologist tells you that it isn't. ∎

NEW FINDING

Box 3-14: Picato Gel effective in clearing actinic keratosis within 2-3 days

A study of 900 actinic keratosis (AK) patients conducted at Mount Sinai School of Medicine suggests that Picato Gel (ingenol mebutate) is an effective treatment. The subjects were randomly assigned to either a Picato or placebo group. When used on the face or scalp, the experimental substance (Picato Gel) cleared the condition about 43 percent of the time, compared to four percent for the control group. For use on the trunk or extremities, the gel was effective 34 percent of the time, compared to approximately five percent for the placebo users. The authors of the study concluded that ingenol mebutate gel applied for two to three days was effective for treatment of AK. The gel appears to be unique in that it takes a relatively short period of time to clear the condition.

(*New England Journal of Medicine,* March 15, 2012)

4 OTHER CONDITIONS

Changes in the skin become more visible with age, and some of those changes are due to conditions and diseases that need medical attention. This chapter describes the skin conditions you are most likely to encounter. The information will make you aware of the symptoms, outline treatment options, and suggest ways to avoid the problems or to prevent a recurrence once they have been treated or cured.

Aging skin

> **WHAT YOU SHOULD KNOW ABOUT...**
>
> **Aging skin**
> - Up to 50 percent of Americans who live to age 65 will have skin cancer at least once.
> - Not exercising regularly contributes to aging skin because exercise promotes muscle tone and increases circulation.
> - With repeated exposure to the sun, the skin loses the ability to repair itself.
> - Wounds take longer to heal.
> - Melanocytes (cells that produce pigment) cluster in areas exposed to the sun, resulting in brown spots (liver or age spots).

The first thing most people notice about natural (intrinsic) aging is wrinkles. They develop when collagen and elastin, the two components that maintain skin firmness, begin to weaken. Instead of remaining thick and tight, the skin becomes thin and loose.

The other natural aging conditions include thinner and more transparent skin, the loss of fat underneath the top layers of skin, sagging skin due to bone loss, dry skin, easily bruised skin, difficulty in cooling the skin by perspiration, hair that turns gray or white, loss of hair, and unwanted hair (in the outer ears, for example). Aging skin has a genetic component, which is why some people get gray hair in their 20s or begin to lose their hair much earlier in life than others. Box 4-1 lists some skin changes that can occur with age.

Gravity is an example of extrinsic, or external, aging. It takes a toll, constantly pulling downward on our skin. The age varies from person to person, but skin elasticity declines dramatically during one's 50s. The tip of the nose might droop, earlobes get longer, eyelids seem to fall, jowls develop, and the upper lip tends to disappear while the lower lip is more pronounced—not a comforting thought, but it's a normal part of aging.

According to the American Academy of Dermatology (AAD), sleep lines can result from lying in the same position every night and resting the face the same way on the pillow. These wrinkles eventually become part of the face's landscape, even when not sleeping or resting. Women tend to get them on their cheeks and chin, while men are more likely to see them on the forehead. The solution, if it's not too late, is to sleep on your back and prevent the skin from bunching up against a pillow.

Smoking accelerates skin aging. People who smoke at least 10 cigarettes a day for 10 years are more likely to develop wrinkles than nonsmokers. Smokers' skin also may have a yellowish hue. Although wrinkles in the face are not visible until later in life, they can be seen under a microscope in smokers still in their 20s. But it's never too late to quit smoking and to reverse or at least slow down the wrinkling process.

Don't believe what you hear or see about facial exercises to avoid wrinkles. They might even cause more fine lines and wrinkles. As skin ages, the loss of elasticity restricts its ability to spring back to its original wrinkle-free state. Save the exercises for other parts of the body.

The sun is, by far, the most damaging external aging factor. Relatively little exposure can cause freckles, "liver spots," spider veins, leathery skin, wrinkles, loose skin, a blotchy complexion, reddish patches, and skin cancer, says the AAD.

Photoaging is the technical term for exposure to the sun, and the amount of photoaging is determined by skin color and the length of long-term exposure. The skin normally can heal itself after overexposure, but with age it loses that ability. The damaging effects appear at a much earlier age if you don't protect your skin. Photoaging is visible using special cameras years before it becomes apparent to you or others.

BOX 4-1: SKIN CHANGES AND POSSIBLE CAUSES

CHANGES	POSSIBLE CAUSES
Sagging skin	Loss of elastin and collagen
Transparent skin	Thinning of the epidermis
Fragile skin	Flattening of the epidermis and dermis
Bruised skin	Thinner blood vessel walls
Itching, dry skin	Loss of sweat and oil glands; overheated indoor air
Sleep lines	Sleeping with your face in the same position over time
Liver spots	Long-term exposure to sunlight
Jowls, double chin	Gravity
Yellowish color	Smoking

Hyaluronic acid is one of many substances applied on top of the skin or injected to lessen the effects of wrinkles, dark spots, fine lines, and other age-related skin conditions. Injections with dermal fillers that contain hyaluronic acid may stimulate the production of collagen, a protein that can partially restore the structure of skin damaged by sunlight. The injections, in effect, "stretch" the cells and allow the collagen to fill the space.

Topical retinol is another option. Non-commercialized lotions containing retinol appear to significantly reduce wrinkles, roughness, and overall aging severity. Retinol, as well as carbon dioxide laser resurfacing (which uses high-intensity light to rejuvenate wrinkled skin), improves overall skin appearance by stimulating the production of collagen. One study found that "wrinkle scores" improved by up to 45 percent among a group of patients who underwent carbon dioxide laser resurfacing.

Alpha-hydroxy acids (AHAs), derived from fruit and milk sugars, are contained in many cosmetics. Although these products are safe in most cases, the U.S. Food and Drug Administration (FDA) has received reports from consumers regarding adverse reactions, including redness, swelling around the eyes, burning sensations, blistering, bleeding, rashes, itching, and skin discoloration. The National Women's Health Information Center (NWHIC) suggests that consumers check the list of ingredients on the outer labels of cosmetics. A listing is required by law. AHAs may be listed by other names, such as glycolic acid and lactic acid. The NWHIC recommends buying and using only products with an AHA level of 10 percent or less, as well as protecting your skin with a 15 or higher SPF sunscreen. You should be doing that even if you're not using a cosmetic product with AHA. Box 4-2 lists selected skin care substances, how they are administered, and the problems they target.

Age spots (liver spots) are caused by long-term exposure to the sun. They are larger than freckles and usually appear in older adults on the face, hands, arms, back, and feet. They may be accompanied by wrinkling, dryness, thinning of the skin, and rough spots. Several over-the-counter products claim to fade age spots, but a prescription drug recommended by a dermatologist and used for several months is more likely to provide lasting results.

Aging and drying skin can cause itching and flaking, especially for those who live in cold, dry, or windy areas. Moisturizers (petrolatum is an example) applied right after bathing can minimize dry skin. Other

BOX 4-2: SKIN CARE SUBSTANCES, METHOD OF ADMINISTRATION, AND PURPOSE

NAME	METHOD OF ADMINISTRATION	PROBLEMS/ AREAS TARGETED
Retinol	Topical cream, lotion	Dark spots, fine lines, wrinkles
Alpha-hydroxy acid	Topical cream, lotion	Skin color, fine lines, age spots
Beta-hydroxy acid	Topical cream	Skin texture, color, acne
Hydroquinone	Topical cream	Dark spots, age spots
Kojic acid	Topical cream	Brown skin pigment/color
Alpha-lipoic acid	Topical lotion, cream	Fine lines, skin tone
Hyaluronic acid	Injected	Wrinkles
Collagen	Injected	Wrinkles
Botulinum toxin	Injected	Wrinkles

moisturizers contain chemicals (urea, AHA, lactic acid, and ammonium lactate) that reduce scaling and assist the skin in holding water. Some, however, can irritate the skin. Ask your dermatologist for help on deciding which moisturizer is best for your age and skin type.

Age- and illness-related skin care

The American Geriatrics Society offers a list of basic skin care tips for older Americans who have age-related skin conditions or illnesses. Some of the suggestions reinforce basic tips described in Chapter 2, some have a slightly different approach or emphasis for this age group, and some apply only to those who have a skin condition or disease.

Dry, itchy skin

1. After a shower or bath, pat your skin gently with a towel, but leave the skin moist. Then apply a lotion, body oil, or moisturizer that is high in petroleum (Aquaphor or Eucerin).
2. Take fewer showers and baths, and use good bathing techniques. Don't scrub the skin roughly. Use a cloth or sponge instead of a rough washcloth. Use a soap containing glycerin or one that has a moisturizing cream, like Dove or Tone.
3. Change bed sheets and clothing often. Wash clothes and sheets in detergents free of perfumes and fabric softeners that could irritate the skin.

4. Drink lots of fluids, and avoid or minimize caffeine and alcohol.
5. Use a humidifier to keep the air moist. Change the water every day to limit the growth of bacteria.

Fungal infections
1. Keep skin clean and dry.
2. Change socks and shoes once a day.
3. Wear loose cotton clothing.
4. Use antifungal powders or creams, such as clotrimazole (Lotrimin) or miconazole (Micatin). Apply the cream to the affected area, and then sprinkle the antifungal powder over the cream.

Voriconazole is a prescription drug used to treat serious fungal infections. Approximately two percent of those who use the drug develop skin reactions such as photo-sensitivity. One study found that five cases of non-invasive melanoma were associated with long-term use of voriconazole.

Shingles
1. When blisters break, keep the area of skin clean and dry until it heals.
2. Take acetaminophen (Tylenol, Excedrin) or other over-the-counter pain medications to relieve symptoms.
3. For more severe episodes, your doctor may prescribe acyclovir (Zovirax), valacyclovir (Valtrex), or famciclovir (Famvir).
4. Ask your doctor or nurse about a dressing to cover sensitive areas.

Pressure sores (when caring for a patient confined to a bed, chair, or wheelchair)
1. Change positions every one to two hours to maintain good
2. blood flow.
3. Keep sheets pulled flat (without wrinkles).
4. Encourage the patient to stand, walk, or perform mild exercises that involve the arms and legs (modified push-ups, for example, when sitting in a wheelchair). These activities increase blood circulation, which helps prevent and heal pressure sores.
5. Keep skin clean and dry.
6. Do not use coated plastic materials that cause sweating under
7. the patient.
8. Gently massage the skin, but not around red areas.

9. Use pads or protectors on heels and elbows.
10. Encourage the patient to eat a varied diet with adequate protein (four to six ounces of meat or fish) and to take a multivitamin that contains zinc and magnesium.

Psoriasis

> **WHAT YOU SHOULD KNOW ABOUT...**
>
> **Psoriasis**
> - Psoriasis is an inflammatory disease of the skin.
> - 150,000 new cases are reported each year.
> - Men and women are equally susceptible.
> - Psoriasis is treatable, but not curable.

Psoriasis is a chronic, inflammatory, immune-related condition of the skin that affects between five million and eight million people in the United States—150,000 new cases every year. An estimated 40 percent of psoriasis patients do not get treatment.

Men and women are equally susceptible. Caucasians are affected more often than African-Americans, and for older adults, peak onset occurs between ages 50 and 60. There are five types of psoriasis, and each has unique symptoms, but 80 percent of people get the most common variety: plaque psoriasis.

A study published in the May 4, 2012 issue of the *American Journal of Human Genetics* identified the first gene directly linked to plaque psoriasis. The discovery of a mutation in the CARD14 gene suggests that it plus an environmental trigger is enough to cause psoriasis. According to the authors of the study, "We now have a much clearer picture of what is happening in psoriasis, and the field is wide open to find new therapeutic targets."

Approximately one-third of psoriasis patients have a family history of the disease. It develops when T cells that normally protect the body against infection and disease develop and rise to the surface at a faster-than-normal rate (see Box 4-3). They accumulate on the top layer of skin before they have time to mature. Skin cell turnover usually takes about a month, but in psoriasis it can happen in a few days. This process results in patches of thick, inflamed skin covered with scales that itch and can hurt. They can appear anywhere on the body, but show up most often on the

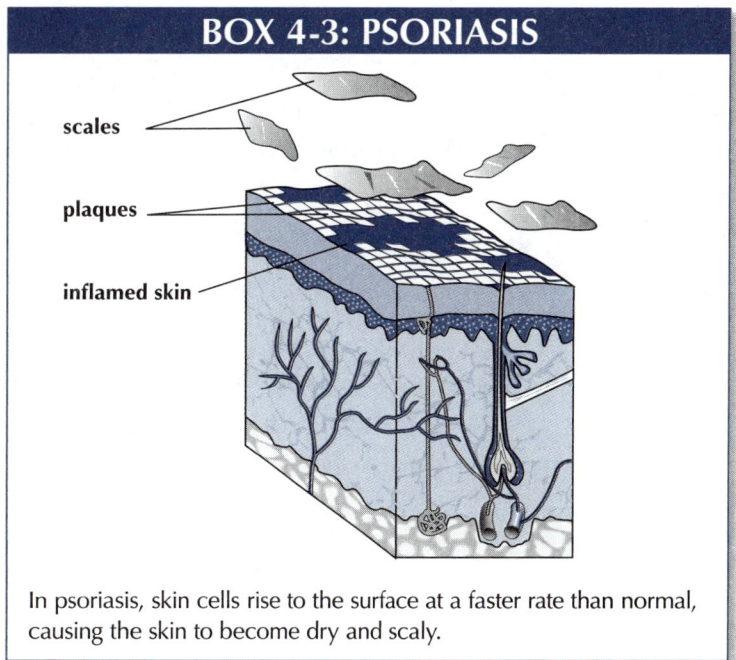

BOX 4-3: PSORIASIS

In psoriasis, skin cells rise to the surface at a faster rate than normal, causing the skin to become dry and scaly.

elbows, knees, legs, lower back, face, palms, soles of the feet, and scalp. The symptoms can be merely a nuisance or serious enough to interfere with work, recreation, and daily functions.

Symptoms also come and go, with varying levels of severity. They include red patches, silver scales, dry skin, cracked skin that can bleed, thick or ridged nails, and swollen or stiff joints. A new episode can be triggered by infections, injuries to the skin, smoking, cold temperatures, stress, alcohol consumption, and certain medications, including lithium, beta blockers, and antimalarial drugs. Excessive body weight can increase the risk of psoriasis.

Information presented at the March 16, 2012 meeting of the American Academy of Dermatology confirmed that excessive inflammation is a critical feature of psoriasis. Inflammation is also a characteristic of insulin resistance, obesity, high cholesterol levels, and cardiovascular disease. Psoriasis patients and their health care providers should watch closely for signs of these diseases.

"1-2-3" treatment

Psoriasis can look like other skin diseases and can be difficult to diagnose. It is not curable, but it is treatable. See a doctor if the condition is more than a nuisance, if it interferes with daily activities, and if you are concerned about the appearance of your skin. If your doctor cannot make a diagnosis by observation, he or she will take a skin sample and examine it under a microscope. Once psoriasis is diagnosed, physicians often use a "1-2-3" approach to treatment.

Step 1 is to prescribe or recommend a topical medication, which could include any of the following substances:

- **Corticosteroids** (reduce inflammation and slow cell turnover)
- **Calcipotriene** (a synthetic form of vitamin D that limits cell production)
- **Retinoids** (synthetic forms of vitamin A that normalize DNA activity in cells)
- **Moisturizers** (reduce itching, scaling and drying)

Combinations of topical drugs are more effective than any single topical application alone.

Step 2 is phototherapy, or the use of natural or artificial ultraviolet (UV) light. When UV light is absorbed into the skin, it can affect the production of T cells and slow the rate of turnover that causes the scaling effect. Limited exposure to sunlight may improve psoriasis, but overexposure can make symptoms worse and damage the skin. Talk to your doctor about the safest use of natural sunlight. Phototherapy can also be combined with other therapies, such as application of a retinoid substance or coal tar ointments.

Step 3 is taking drugs by injection or orally that treat the body's entire immune system (systemic therapy). Drugs used to treat more severe forms of psoriasis may produce serious side effects, such as nausea, dizziness, bruising, fatigue, and kidney malfunction. These drugs include:

- Methotrexate (suppresses the immune system)
- Retinoids (used when other treatment fails)
- Cyclosporine (suppresses the immune system)
- 6-Thioguanine (suppresses the immune system)
- Hydroxyurea (sometimes combined with other treatments)
- Antibiotics (sometimes used when an infection triggers psoriasis)
- Biologics (drugs made from human or animal protein that block the effects of cells that cause inflammation)

Biologics include Amevive, Enbrel, Humira, Raptiva, and Remicade. These drugs, according to the National Psoriasis Foundation, are better at targeting overactive immune cells (specifically T cells) and produce fewer side effects than other psoriasis drugs. Biologics have to be administered by injection or by intravenous infusion. The latter can take up to two hours. They appear to be a safe treatment option for people with psoriasis and psoriatic arthritis, but their long-term effects are not known. Also, they should not be prescribed for a person who is already taking another drug that suppresses the immune system.

Researchers at universities in Pennsylvania and Utah found that biologics are only marginally better than standard treatment and considerably more expensive. Nevertheless, some dermatologists think that this class of drugs gives patients reason to hope for better outcomes (see Box 4-4).

Other types of drugs are promising. A class of diabetes drugs known as thiazoli-dinediones (TZDs) may reduce the risk of psoriasis. A drug (alefacept) that reduces the activity of immune cells is effective for the treatment of scalp psoriasis. And, low-dose treatment with acitretin may minimize the effects of nail psoriasis.

Self-care

The Mayo Clinic suggests the following ways you can treat, but not cure, psoriasis:

NEW FINDING

Box 4-4: Mixed outcomes for new psoriasis drugs

New and more expensive psoriasis medications called biologics are marginally better than the standard methotrexate treatment, according to researchers at the University of Pennsylvania and University of Utah. A study of 713 patients, conducted over a year-and-a-half period, showed that improvement ranged from 24 percent among methotrexate users to between 34 and 48 percent among subjects who received biologics. However, biologics can cost up to $20,000 a year, compared to about $2,000 per year for methotrexate. The study also showed that phototherapy was generally as effective as methotrexate, but inconvenient because patients must get treatment three times a week for three months and dangerous because it raises the risk of skin cancer. In spite of the negative news, some dermatologists think that biologics give patients hope where there was previously no hope.

(*Archives of Dermatology*, April 2012)

- Daily baths to remove scales and reduce inflammation (but avoid hot water and harsh soaps).
- Moisturizers to prevent drying of the skin.
- Covering affected areas at night (moisturizers wrapped with plastic).
- Cortisone to reduce inflammation (over-the-counter creams containing 0.5 to one percent cortisone).
- Avoiding triggers (stress, smoking, excessive sun exposure and alcohol).

Tips for psoriasis patients from the ADA
- Eat a balanced diet.
- Stay physically active.
- Don't smoke; limit alcohol consumption.
- Maintain ideal weight.
- Reduce stress.
- Get regular checks for cardiovascular risk factors.
- Control blood pressure, blood sugar, and cholesterol.

Psoriatic arthritis

Between 10 and 30 percent of people who have psoriasis develop a condition called psoriatic arthritis. Not everyone who has psoriasis develops psoriatic arthritis, but all of those diagnosed with psoriatic arthritis have psoriasis. It can develop at any age, but is seen most often in adults between ages 30 and 50. Genes, environmental factors, and the immune system appear to play a role in the development of psoriatic arthritis, which affects men slightly more often than women. Psoriasis precedes psoriatic arthritis by months or even years.

The symptoms are pain and stiffness in the knees, ankles, and joints of the feet, although other areas can be affected. The inflamed joints may be swollen and hot, and stiffness and pain are worse in the morning than at other times. Patients also may have inflamed tendons and inflammation in the eyes, lungs, and aorta. Acne is a common side effect.

Diagnosing psoriatic arthritis is done with X-rays, joint fluid tests, and blood tests. Treatment is aimed at suppressing the symptoms rather than curing the disease. Doctors usually try nonsteroidal anti-inflammatory drugs (NSAIDs), such as aspirin and ibuprofen, first. If they don't work, disease-modifying antirheumatic drugs (DMARDs), such as methotrexate, antimalarials, sulfasalazine, cyclosporine, and tumor necrosis factor (TNF) inhibitors, are prescribed. TNF drugs, such as etanercept (Enbrel), infliximab (Remicade), and adalimumab (Humira), are effective for psoriasis and psoriatic arthritis.

The FDA has approved the drugs golimumab (trade name Simponi) and ustekinumab (Stelara) for the treatment of psoriatic arthritis.

If arthritis is the focus, a rheumatologist should treat it. Psoriasis as a skin disease requires only treatment by a dermatologist.

Shingles

> **WHAT YOU SHOULD KNOW ABOUT...**
>
> **Shingles**
> - One-third of Americans will develop shingles sooner or later.
> - Most people who get shingles are over age 60.
> - A gene has been identified that is directly linked to plaque psoriasis.
> - Shingles occurs only in people who have had chickenpox.
> - The Centers for Diseases Control and Prevention recommends a shingles vaccination for adults over the age of 60.

A third of Americans will suffer from shingles at some point, and the majority of them will be over age 60. During any given year, one million people in the United States alone develop the disease.

Shingles is caused by the herpes zoster virus, the same one that causes chickenpox. In fact, people who get chickenpox as children retain the dormant virus in nerve cells. Later in life, the virus can reemerge for unknown reasons. Shingles itself develops only from a reactivation of the virus in someone who previously had chickenpox. Those who are most susceptible are age 50 and older, are under stress, are ill, and have a weakened immune system because of age, disease, or medications. Family history also might make a person more susceptible to shingles.

Shingles is not contagious, but the virus that causes it can be spread by direct contact from a person who has the condition to another person who has not had chickenpox. That person will get chickenpox, not shingles.

The two distinguishing symptoms of shingles are a skin rash on one side of the trunk, and pain. The first sign may be a burning or tingling sensation, itching, or numbness. After a few days, a rash of blisters filled with fluid may appear as a band covering one side of the trunk from the back to the front of the body and downward to the waistline, but shingles can also affect the face and eyes. The pain associated with shingles can be mild or severe, but don't underestimate its severity when people complain about it. The slightest touch or contact can cause excruciating pain.

The blisters normally last a week to 10 days, then form a crust and fall off. In some cases, this process can take three to five weeks. The

> **NEW FINDING**
>
> **Box 4-5: Shingles vaccine safe and has few side effects**
>
> A study of 193,083 adults age 50 and older found that the herpes zoster vaccine, also known as the shingles vaccine, does not increase the risk of stroke, heart disease, infection of the brain, Bell's palsy, or Ramsay-Hunt syndrome. Researchers found a small increased risk of local reactions (redness and pain) from one to seven days after the vaccination. The study supports the CDC's recommendation and reassures that the vaccine is safe. Zostavax, the trade name for the vaccine, was approved by the FDA in 2006 for use in healthy people over the age of 60.
>
> (*Journal of Internal Medicine*, published online April 22, 2012)

skin may change color (darker) once the rash subsides. Although the rash improves, the pain can last longer. Twenty percent of those who get shingles develop a condition known as postherpetic neuralgia (PHN)—nerve pain without the rash that can persist for years. The older you are when you get shingles, the more likely you are to develop PHN. The main symptom is pain so severe that it can cause insomnia, weight loss, and depression.

Treatment

There is no cure for shingles, but the symptoms can be greatly relieved by taking anti-viral drugs such as acyclovir (Zovirax), famciclovir (Famvir), or valacyclovir (Val-trex). Other medications used to treat symptoms are steroids, anticonvulsants, antidepressants, and over-the-counter pain medications such as acetaminophen (Tylenol) and ibuprofen (Advil, Motrin). A medicated lotion such as Benadryl or Caladryl might reduce the pain and itching, as will cool compresses soaked in an astringent liquid (Bluboro, Domeboro).

Although shingles is incurable, it may be preventable. The U.S. Centers for Disease Control and Prevention recommends that adults over age 60 get a single dose of the shingles vaccine Zostavax, which has been approved by the FDA. The vaccine has cut the projected number of shingles cases by half, and in those who are infected despite the shots, the severity and complications (including postherpetic neuralgia) are significantly reduced.

A study of more than 190,000 adults over the age of 50 published in the *Journal of Internal Medicine* found that the shingles vaccine is safe and has few side effects. It does not, contrary to earlier reports, increase the risk of heart disease, stroke, infection of the brain, Bell's palsy, or Ramsay-Hunt syndrome (see Box 4-5).

However, Zostavax is not for everyone. Those who have a weakened immune system should not get the vaccination. Ask your doctor if a vaccination is appropriate for your age and medical condition.

Diabetes-related skin conditions

About 33 percent of people who have diabetes will have a diabetes-related skin problem, according to the American Diabetes Association (ADA). Sometimes, the skin disorder is the first sign that diabetes is present.

The warm, high-sugar content of the body's blood is a perfect environment for the growth and development of skin-related bacterial and fungal infections. Anyone can get these skin conditions, but diabetics are more susceptible.

A common symptom of many skin diseases is itching (also called pruritus). It can be caused by a variety of things, including dry skin, yeast infections, or diminished blood flow to an area of the skin. Lower legs are affected more often than other regions of the body. Lotions and moisturizers can limit itching by keeping the skin soft and moist, but in excessive amounts applied to certain areas, they can provide an environment conducive to infections.

Bacterial infections

Styes, boils, carbuncles, and nail infections are examples of bacterial infections that can occur in people with diabetes. The symptoms are hot, swollen, red, and painful spots at different areas, depending on the condition (styes on the eyelids; boils around hair follicles; carbuncles deep in the skin; nail infections on hands or feet). The most common type of bacterial infection is staphylococcus—"staph," for short.

Bacterial infections are treatable with antibiotics and perhaps preventable by controlling blood sugar levels. Nevertheless, diabetics are affected more than non-diabetics, and only a doctor can diagnose the infection and prescribe medications—either in pill or cream form.

Fungal infections

Athlete's foot, jock itch, ringworm, and vaginal infections are fungal infections that affect the general population, but which present special problems for people with diabetes. The cause is often Candida albicans (CA), a yeast-like fungus that targets diabetics. It causes an itchy, red area surrounded by small blisters and scales, usually in warm, moist folds of the skin such as the mouth, vagina, breasts, fingers, toes, nails, and rectum. CA can move through the bloodstream and affect distant areas of the body.

Other diabetes-related conditions

Four problems—diabetic dermopathy, necrobiosis lipoidica, diabetic blisters, and eruptive xanthomatosis—are either specific to people who have diabetes or occur most frequently in those who have the disease.

Diabetic dermopathy

Diabetic dermopathy is caused by changes in small blood vessels that result in light brown, scaly, oval or circular patches of skin, usually on the front of the legs. The patches do not itch, hurt, or drain. They are generally harmless and do not require treatment.

Necrobiosis lipoidica (NL)
Necrobiosis lipoidica diabeticorum is a rare condition caused by a change in the blood vessels, and consists of oval plaques, usually on the lower legs. It is similar to diabetic dermopathy, but the spots are larger, deeper, and fewer in number. NL may begin as small red or raised spots, which develop a shiny appearance surrounded by a violet-colored border. The spots often turn brown and fade, but usually leave a permanent discoloration. NL can be painful and can itch. Adult women are the most likely victims, and diabetics account for two-thirds of all cases. If the plaques break open, see a dermatologist for treatment.

Diabetic blisters
In rare cases, people can develop diabetic blisters on their fingers, hands, toes, feet, legs, or forearms. They resemble blisters caused by burns, but are not painful. Diabetic blisters normally heal in two to three weeks without treatment. Those who develop the blisters often suffer diabetic neuropathy, a nerve disorder caused by diabetes. The only way to guard against the incidence of diabetic blisters is to keep blood sugar levels under control.

Eruptive xanthomatosis (EX)
Eruptive xanthomatosis is a problem when diabetes has gotten out of control. The symptoms are small, firm, yellow bumps on the skin. A red circle surrounds the bumps, and the area may itch. EX usually appears on the backs of hands, feet, arms, legs, and buttocks. A person at risk has type 1 diabetes and elevated blood lipids (fats). Once the person's blood sugar level is brought back to acceptable levels, the bumps disappear.

Prevention
The ADA suggests the following measures to prevent or reduce the risk of diabetes-related skin diseases:
- Keep skin clean and dry by using talcum powder where skin touches skin.
- Avoid hot baths, hot showers, and putting lotion between your toes. Warm, moist surfaces are breeding grounds for infections.

- Prevent dry skin (which can crack and allow microorganisms to get in) by using moisturizers, especially in cold, windy weather.
- Treat cuts immediately. Wash them with soap and water, but avoid products that are too harsh, such as alcohol and iodine. Use antibiotic cream only if approved by your doctor.
- Keep your home more humid than normal during cold, dry months. Bathe less, if practical.
- Use mild shampoos, and avoid feminine hygiene sprays.
- See a dermatologist for skin conditions you cannot treat successfully.

Boils

The type of boil familiar to most people begins as a red, elevated, warm, and painful bump on the skin, often caused by an infected hair follicle. Later, the area may get bigger, softer, and even more painful. Individuals with diabetes, immune deficiencies, poor nutrition, and poor hygiene are at a greater risk for boils than the general population. The condition is caused by bacteria, and a staphylococcus infection is often the culprit.

Boils can develop anywhere on the body, but common sites are the face, neck, armpits, buttocks, groin, and thighs. In addition to an infected hair follicle, boils can be triggered by ingrown hair, a foreign object imbedded in the skin, a plugged sweat gland, or blocked oil duct. Within a week, the area turns white as pus makes its way to the surface. Sometimes, it drains through the skin. At other times, it has to be lanced and drained by a physician. Several boils can develop at the same time because the infection spreads to the surrounding area or is transported to some other part of the body.

Treatment

Self-care includes applying warm compresses or soaking the boil in warm water for 20 minutes, three or four times a day. The increase in temperature draws the pus closer to the surface of the skin, and it may make the area less painful. Putting antibiotic creams on the area before the boil comes to a head won't work, because the medicine does not penetrate the skin. "Coming to a head" means the top of the area breaks and the pus drains out, but the process could take as long as 10 days.

Do not lance the boil yourself, as doing so could allow the infection to spread. If and when the boil does break, keep the area clean by gently washing it with an antibacterial soap two or three times a day. Apply a medicated ointment and cover the area with a bandage.

See a doctor if the infected area seems to be getting worse, if you develop a fever, if the boil does not drain, if additional boils appear, if the boil limits your normal activities, or if you have diabetes. Don't take chances. If in doubt, call your family doctor or a dermatologist.

Prevention

There are no guarantees, but you might be able to prevent boils by:
- Keeping boil-prone areas clean
- Not sharing towels, clothes, and linens with a family member or friend who has a boil
- Immediately cleaning and treating minor cuts and scrapes
- Not wearing clothes that fit too tightly

Cysts

Sebaceous, epidermoid, epidermal, and keratin are all terms used in various medical publications to describe small, fairly common cysts that develop just below the surface of the skin.

True sebaceous cysts are less common than epidermoid cysts, and the growths are associated with sebaceous glands, not hair follicles, which usually give rise to more common epidermoid cysts. The word "keratin" is used because common kinds of cysts are filled with an oily protein called keratin.

The National Institutes of Health refers to them as epidermal cysts, and that is what they will be called here. But it is more important to understand what cysts are and what, if anything, should be done about them.

Epidermal cysts are sacs beneath the surface of the skin filled with keratin and fatty material. They often develop at the site of a damaged hair follicle on the face, neck, trunk, genital area, and behind the ears. In some cases, there is an opening in the center through which the foul-smelling contents can escape. The fatty content of the cyst causes the odor.

Cysts can be moved around (under the skin) within a small area. They don't hurt, and they don't grow rapidly, but they can become tender, inflamed, and perhaps larger than when you first noticed them. Typical epidermal cysts range in size from a quarter-inch to two inches. When inflammation is involved, cysts are likely to be tender and red, and the temperature of the skin on top of the growth may rise.

The risk factors are age (most people get them during their 30s or 40s), gender (men are twice as likely to get them as women), a history of acne, an injury to the skin (any type of crushing or traumatic injury), and long-term sun exposure.

Treatment

Epidermal cysts are not dangerous and usually require no treatment. If you think one has become inflamed or if you have one that is large enough or painful enough to interfere with daily activities, your doctor can diagnose the condition with a quick examination. In some cases, a biopsy can rule out more serious skin conditions.

A warm compress might help drain the cyst—do not force the drainage yourself—or the doctor might inject the area with a steroid to reduce inflammation. On rare occasions, surgery is required to remove it. Cysts may recur.

You cannot prevent these growths, but avoiding excessive exposure to the sun and using skin products that do not contain oils might help.

Dermatitis

There are more rashes in this world than there is space to describe all of them in this report. Most rashes and skin irritations are triggered by coming into contact with foreign substances. The one that is most likely to cause problems in older adults is dermatitis, and two varieties—allergic contact dermatitis and irritant contact dermatitis—will be discussed here.

A third form is called atopic dermatitis (atopic eczema), which is a condition passed from parents to children that can develop at any time during a person's life, but it is primarily a problem for infants and children. Corticosteroids are still the treatment of choice, but newer, effective gels, foams, and oils have been approved by the FDA.

Allergic contact dermatitis

This rash appears when the immune system overreacts to allergens like poison ivy, poison oak, poison sumac (all of which contain an oily irritant called urushiol), cosmetics, latex, nickel, and hair dyes. Even the fragrances in soaps, shampoos, and perfumes can cause a reaction. Antibodies from your immune system come into contact with the allergens and set off "mediators," such as histamine, which cause the symptoms. Allergic contact dermatitis may appear almost immediately or a day or two after exposure. Symptoms include reddish skin or a rash, an itching or burning sensation, swelling, and blisters that ooze, break, and leave crusts or scales.

Researchers at the University of Mississippi are working on a product that would control the allergic reaction in people already sensitive to poison plants and would prevent it altogether in those who are not sensitive. The product contains chemical derivatives of urushiol, the oily substance in poison ivy, oak, and sumac that causes skin to become inflamed. Clinical trials should begin soon.

Drugs to treat bacterial infections may cause problems themselves. One example is neomycin, a commonly sold over-the-counter antibiotic. In some people it can cause contact dermatitis.

Irritant contact dermatitis

A foreign substance that comes into direct contact with your skin and damages the area causes this form of dermatitis. Cleaning products, such as detergents and solvents, are examples. These irritants can wear down the skin's protective surface. The longer the substance stays on the skin, the more serious the damage, and it could take up to four weeks for the area to return to normal. Symptoms include swelling, a tight feeling in the affected area (hands are often exposed first), dry skin, blisters, ulcers, and skin that itches, cracks, or burns.

Treatment

You can treat itching and other symptoms of most rashes at home with cortisone-based creams to reduce inflammation, calamine lotions, oral antihistamines, and oatmeal baths. Over-the-counter drugs like Benadryl and Ben-Allergin (both of which contain diphenhydramine) also might be effective. It's easier said than done, but don't scratch. In the case of irritant contact dermatitis, wash the area with soap and cool water immediately after contact to get rid of the foreign substance. Treat blisters with cold, moist compresses 30 minutes at a time, three times a day. Get medical help if the rash doesn't improve within two or three days or if it continues to spread.

Prevention

For both allergic and irritant contact dermatitis, the first line of prevention is to identify the source and avoid contact with it. Learn to recognize poison ivy, poison oak, and poison sumac (see Boxes 4-6 and 4-7).

To protect against potential irritants, wear cotton gloves under rubber gloves for protection against wet substances. Use mild soaps that don't irritate the skin, and use hand creams and moisturizers.

Calluses and corns

Although calluses and corns may require attention, neither is a serious problem. Both conditions are areas where the skin has hardened and thickened, both are caused by pressure or friction, and both can develop on the hands or feet. Neither condition is likely to cause pain or tenderness.

Calluses can be more than an inch in diameter. They can develop under the big toes, balls and heels of the feet, on the knees, and on the hands, usually at the base of the fingers. Calluses can actually protect hands and feet under conditions that involve constant friction, such as gardening, farming, and playing a sport.

Corns are smaller than calluses and could have either a hard or soft center. The most likely spot for a soft corn is between the toes, but a hard corn may be on the top or outer sides of the toes.

Neither condition needs treatment unless it causes pain. One way to treat corns and calluses is to avoid the contact that causes friction in the first place or, in the case of the hands, to wear protective gloves. Another is to relieve the pressure by using a doughnut-shaped pad on the foot, and a third is to soften the area with an over-the-counter salicylic acid product before removing the dead skin. In rare cases, surgery is needed to remove a corn or callus.

You shouldn't cut a callus or corn yourself, especially if you have diabetes or any other condition that affects circulation, but you can gradually wear down the area with a pumice stone.

Prevention is always better than treatment, and could include not wearing tight, high-heeled, or loose-fitting shoes, or socks that don't fit. Walking barefoot can also cause calluses and should be avoided when doing so is the cause.

BOX 4-6

How to identify poison ivy, oak, and sumac

Poison ivy:

- Grows as a vine in the East, Midwest, and South, and as a shrub in the West, far North, and Canada
- Each leaf has three leaflets

Poison oak:

- Grows as a vine in the West and a shrub in the East
- Has three leaves or leaflets

Poison sumac:

- Grows in standing water peat bogs in the Northeast and Midwest and in swampy areas of the Southeast
- Each leaf contains seven to 13 leaflets, arranged in paired rows

BOX 4-7: POISON IVY, OAK, AND SUMAC

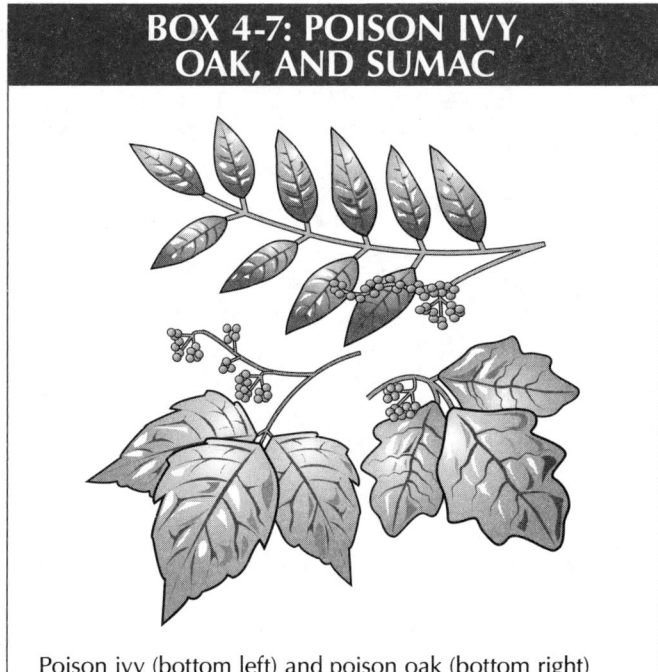

Poison ivy (bottom left) and poison oak (bottom right) have three leaves or leaflets. Poison sumac (top) has leaflets arranged in paired rows.

Skin tags (acrochordon)

> **WHAT YOU SHOULD KNOW ABOUT...**
>
> **Skin tags**
> - They cannot be prevented and are benign, but may be unsightly.
> - A dermatologist can remove them in an office visit.
> - They occur most frequently around the neck, upper chest, shoulders, armpits, and other areas where the skin folds.
> - They can be irritated when something repeatedly rubs against them.
> - They occur most frequently after the age of 60.

A skin tag is one skin condition you won't have to worry about. It is a benign, skin-colored growth that occurs more commonly after age 60. Some skin tags may be darker than the skin color. A tag sticks out of the skin, usually near the neck, armpits, trunk, breasts, or other areas of the body where the skin folds. Tags are small, but some may be up to a half-inch in length.

Skin tags do not grow, they do not hurt, they are not a form of skin cancer, and they don't become skin cancer. The only potential problems are that they are not cosmetically attractive, and they can become irritated if they are in a place where clothes or jewelry rub against them. They may develop because of skin rubbing against skin, and they are more common in those who are overweight or have diabetes.

A skin tag is easily diagnosed and treated. All you or your doctor has to do is look at one to identify it. It can be removed during an office visit by surgery, by freezing it (cryotherapy), or by cauterization (burning it off with an electrical current). Tags do not normally come back at the same site, but new growths can develop elsewhere on the body.

You can't prevent skin tags—they just happen. But unless they regularly become irritated, look unsightly, or change in color, size, composition, or sensitivity, there is no reason to treat or report them.

Seborrheic keratosis

Seborrheic keratosis (SK) can be deceiving. It manifests as a wart-like tumor on the surface of the skin and may be mistaken for skin cancer. It is neither, but SK is a very common skin growth in older adults.

SKs can be yellow, brown, black, or other colors, and they are more common on the face, chest, shoulders, and back than on other places of the body. Some of them turn black, which is why they may be mistaken for skin cancer, but biopsies almost always determine them to be noncancerous. SKs can appear alone or in clusters, have a rough or smooth texture, and do not penetrate deeply into the skin. They can be very small or more than an inch in diameter, and they are painless. However, rubbing or scratching SKs can cause inflammation.

Descriptions of SKs include the term "stuck on" or "pasted on," as if someone dabbed a patch of candle wax onto the skin. They are not contagious, but they do seem to run in families.

The cause is unknown, though the name suggests an oily, waxy substance similar to that produced by sebaceous glands. Expert opinions are mixed as to whether ultraviolet light exposure causes SKs. The American Academy of Dermatology says exposure to sunlight does not seem to be a cause or a complicating factor after SKs have developed. The Mayo Clinic says exposure to sunlight may be a factor because the condition is common in areas often exposed to the sun.

Treatment

The best news about SKs is that they are not dangerous, and usually do not need to be removed. People who do have them taken off do so because of their unsightly appearance or because the growths get irritated, itch, or bleed. Insurance companies do not cover procedures to remove them for cosmetic purposes. If a skin growth similar to an SK develops rapidly, ask a dermatologist to check the area.

Don't waste your money on creams, ointments, or other over-the-counter products that claim to remove the growths. They don't work. A dermatologist can remove an SK during an office visit by cryosurgery (using liquid nitrogen), curettage (scraping them off the skin), electrosurgery (by means of an electrical current, sometimes combined with curettage), or laser surgery (using high-intensity light beams to destroy the growth).

Do not confuse seborrheic keratosis with actinic keratosis. Actinic keratosis, also called solar keratosis, is considered to be the earliest stage of skin cancer that is limited to the outer-most layer of skin.

Rosacea

> **WHAT YOU SHOULD KNOW ABOUT...**
>
> **Rosacea**
> - Rosacea affects 14 million Americans.
> - Family history and sunburns may be associated with rosacea.
> - Most people with rosacea don't know they have it.
> - 78 percent of Americans have never heard of it.
> - Rosacea is treatable and manageable, but not curable.

Rosacea is a fairly common skin disease that affects the face and neck. The symptoms vary from person to person, but the most common signs are redness that resembles a sunburn, small red bumps or pimples that may contain pus, and very small but visible blood vessels on the surface of the skin. The cheeks, forehead, chin, and nose are the primary targets; the neck, ears, chest, and back are less frequently involved. In 50 percent of people with rosacea, the eyes may be watery, red, or irritated. Other possible symptoms are a sensation of burning, itching, or stinging, dry or thick skin, and facial swelling.

Individuals most susceptible to the condition have fair skin, blush easily, are between ages 30 and 60, and have a family history of the condition. Women are affected more often than men, but that may be because men wait longer to seek treatment.

The cause of rosacea is unknown, but recent research revealed that an immune response might play a role in its development. Through skin biopsies, a team of international researchers found that people with rosacea had unusually high levels of cathelicidins (types of proteins), peptides, and inflammatory properties that protect skin against infection. They also discovered that an enzyme known as SCTE was elevated in people with rosacea. Although the research is at a very early stage, it is possible that high levels of these substances, instead of protecting the skin, make certain people more susceptible to rosacea and other skin conditions.

Some experts theorize that rosacea is caused by a disorder of the blood vessels, skin mites, a fungal infection, a malfunction of the connective tissue under the skin, or unspecified psychological factors.

A family history of rosacea places people in a higher risk category, as do high rates of blistering sunburn. The National Rosacea Society (NRS) reports a connection between rosacea and national origin. Individuals with Irish, English, and German ancestry appear to be at especially high risk.

Rosacea has psychological as well as physical consequences. A survey conducted by the NRS found that more than 75 percent of patients said their condition lowered their self-confidence and self-esteem. Fifty-two percent said it was the reason for avoiding public contact and cancelling social engagements.

Treatment

If rosacea is not treated, it always gets worse and sometimes progresses into a more serious condition called rhinophyma, which affects the nose, giving it a red, bulbous appearance. Almost 90 percent of rosacea patients say their condition is under control with treatment. Treatment varies, depending on which symptoms are targeted, and usually consists of a combination approach.

Topical medications include azelaic acid, benzoyl peroxide, clindamycin, erythromycin, metronidazole, sulfacetamide, and sulfur lotions. It might take two or three months to get significant results.

Pimples and bumps may respond better to oral antibiotics, including doxycycline, erythromycin, minocycline, and tetracycline.

Oral antibiotics may be combined with glycolic acid peels and glycolic washes and creams. Isotretinoin is not approved by the FDA for this condition, but some doctors prescribe it (off-label use) to help shrink facial skin that has thickened. However, it has serious side effects, such as nosebleeds, dry skin, dry mouth and itching.

When the eyes are affected, patients should gently clean their eyelids with diluted baby shampoo or an over-the-counter eyelid cleaning substance. Warm compresses applied several times a day might relieve the symptoms. Oral antibiotics such as doxycycline, minocycline, or tetracycline are prescribed at times.

Dermatologists may use electrosurgery or laser surgery to address redness and flushing. Among recent innovations are pulsed dye lasers that destroy visible blood vessels and reduce flushing and redness. Intense pulsed light therapy delivers light to the affected areas, where it targets blood vessels and redness.

Prevention

Rosacea cannot be prevented, but the symptoms can be controlled once they have developed. The first step is to avoid possible triggers, such as exposure to sun and wind, emotionally stressful situations, hot and cold weather extremes, strenuous exercise, alcohol (including cosmetics that contain alcohol), hot beverages, hot baths, and rubbing, scrubbing, or massaging the face.

Use a 15 SPF or higher sunscreen when you will be outdoors, and during winter, prevent dry skin by using a moisturizer. Consider keeping a diary to identify substances, activities, and environments that could cause a flare-up of rosacea.

Sunburn

WHAT YOU SHOULD KNOW ABOUT...

Sunburn
- Most skin diseases are associated with overexposure to the sun.
- Any part of the body can be sunburned, including the eyes.
- A person with light-colored skin can get a sunburn in as little as 15 minutes.
- Older adults are more susceptible to sunburn than young and middle-age adults.
- If your shadow is shorter than you are, you are being exposed to high levels of UV radiation.

Most, if not all, skin diseases are partially or fully caused by overexposure to the sun, and if not caused by the sun, many of them are made worse by exposure to ultraviolet (UV) rays. However, there are benefits to sun exposure, particularly in the case of UV rays helping the body produce vitamin D, which is often lacking in older adults.

The most immediate, short-term problem caused by the sun is sunburn. According to the National Institutes of Health (NIH), sunburn occurs when the amount of exposure to ultraviolet rays, whether from the sun or from artificial sources, exceeds the body's ability to produce melanin. Melanin is a protective pigment responsible for tanning, and a suntan is the body's way of shielding itself against UV rays.

Sunburn is not immediately apparent. Symptoms start to appear about four hours after exposure, get worse during the next six to 48 hours, and begin to subside in three to five days. In a mild case of sunburn, the skin becomes red or pink, warm, and tender. In more severe burns, the symptoms are pain, swollen skin, and possibly blisters. By the time your skin is painful and red, the damage has been done. If a large area is burned, you might experience a headache, fever, nausea, or fatigue. The skin will begin to peel three to eight days after exposure. Total recovery ranges from several days to three weeks.

Any part of the body can be sunburned, including the eyes. Sunburned eyes are red, dry, painful, and gritty-feeling. Long-term effects of chronic exposure to the sun include cataracts and perhaps macular degeneration (an age-related loss of central vision).

Older adults and young children are more susceptible to sunburn than young and middle-age adults. The way a person's skin reacts to the sun depends on skin type, length of exposure, time of day and year, geography, and drugs that person is taking.

Skin type

Of the many factors associated with sunburn, one of the most important is skin type. Several organizations, including the Skin Cancer Foundation, classify skin types from light to dark. Box 4-8 describes skin types, colors, and reactions

BOX 4-8: SKIN TYPES

SKIN TYPE	CHARACTERISTICS	REACTION TO SUN'S RAYS
Type I	Very fair/white skin; blue or green eyes; blond or red hair	Always burns; never tans
Type II	Fair/white skin; blue, hazel, or brown eyes; blond, red, or brown hair	Burns easily; minimal tan
Type III	Darker white skin	Minimal burn; tans slowly
Type IV	Light brown, olive skin	Minimal burn; tans easily
Type V	Brown skin	Rarely burns; tans easily, darkly
Type VI	Dark brown or black skin	Rarely burns; always tans

to the sun's rays. The closer you are to Type I on the scale, the greater your risk of sunburn now and skin cancer later. The darker the skin, the more pigmentation it has to protect itself against the sun.

Length of exposure

A person who is a Type I or Type II can get a sunburn in as little as 15 minutes, while a person with darker skin may be able to tolerate the same amount of exposure for several hours.

Time of day and year

The highest risk for sunburn is between 10 a.m. and 4 p.m., and exposure during the summer months is especially dangerous.

Geography/location

Snow, water, and light-colored sand reflect UV rays and increase the chances that you will suffer a sunburn. Clouds don't help, as up to 90 percent of UV rays penetrate cloud cover. The higher the elevation and the closer you are to the equator, the greater the risk. The worst possible situation would be swimming or snow-skiing at a high altitude in a country near the equator.

Drugs

Several drugs increase sensitivity to sunlight and the risk of being burned by the sun's rays. Among them are ibuprofen (Motrin, Advil), sulfa antibiotics (Gantanol), doxycycline (Adoxa, Monodox), tetracycline (Periostat, Vibramycin), and diuretics (Diuril, Edecrin).

Treatment

Treatment for sunburn requires patience. There is no quick cure. Aspirin, acetaminophen, and ibuprofen relieve pain and reduce fever. Drink lots of water to replace lost fluid. Cool baths and wet cloths might feel good, as will moisturizing creams. A low-dose (0.5 to one percent) hydrocortisone cream might reduce the burning sensation and hasten the healing process.

If blisters develop, cover the area with a light bandage or gauze. Breaking the blisters will increase the possibility of infection, so allow them to resolve on their own.

See a doctor if more than 15 percent of your body is affected (for example, the upper and lower back, plus the buttocks, constitute 18 percent of your body's skin), if you are dehydrated, if you have a fever exceeding 101 degrees Fahrenheit, or if the pain persists longer than 24 hours.

Prevention

Here are some sunburn-prevention tips provided by the CDC and NIH:

- Use a full-spectrum sunscreen with a minimum 15 SPF and preferably a 30 SPF.
- Apply a sunscreen 20 minutes before being exposed to the sun, and reapply every two hours—sooner if you are in and out of water or if you perspire heavily. There are no waterproof sunscreens.
- Wear dark clothing with a tight weave to block UV rays.
- Wear a wide-brimmed hat that protects the scalp, face, ears, and neck.
- Avoid tanning beds.

Check the UV index on the Internet, in newspapers, or on television weather reports. The index ranges from a low of one to a high of 11. Take extra precautions when the index is high (see Box 4-9).

An easy way to tell how much UV exposure you are getting is to look for your shadow. If your shadow is taller than you are (in the early morning and late afternoon), your UV exposure is likely to be low. If your shadow is shorter than you are (around midday), you are being exposed to high levels of UV radiation. Seek shade and protect your skin and eyes.

Moles (nevi)

Moles are clusters or spots on the skin that consist of melanin cells called melanocytes, which give color to skin. They are usually dark brown, but can be reddish-brown, blue, or the color of skin. They vary in shape and size, but most are oval or round, and most are less than a quarter-inch in diameter. Moles can be flat, raised, smooth, or wrinkled.

Most of us have between 10 and 40 moles, and their presence was probably determined at birth. They can develop on any area of the body, including the scalp, between fingers or toes, and under fingernails and toenails. The number of moles can change with age, some fading as a person moves into adulthood, others disappearing altogether, and some lasting 50 years. Sunlight can increase the number of moles and make them darker, and sunburn may increase the risk of melanoma. People who have the greatest number of moles are at the greatest risk of developing a melanoma.

Most moles are harmless and will never be a threat to a person's health, but certain types carry a higher risk of becoming cancerous. Atypical moles

BOX 4-9: UV INDEX

UV INDEX NUMBER	EXPOSURE LEVEL
2 or less	Low
3 to 5	Moderate
6 to 8	High
9 to 10	Very high
11+	Extreme

(dysplastic nevi) are larger than a pencil eraser and usually have a dark brown center with a lighter, uneven border. They tend to run in families.

Diagnosis and treatment

If you think you have a potentially cancerous mole, see a dermatologist immediately. A biopsy can determine if it is malignant, and a mole can be removed by shave excision (using a small blade to cut it out), punch biopsy (removing the mole with a small device that works like a cookie cutter), and excisional surgery (which involves taking out the mole and the skin around it). All of the procedures can be performed quickly in a dermatologist's office. Once removed, most moles do not recur. If one does, let your doctor know about it.

Prevention

Knowing the early warning signs of melanomas—moles that are asymmetrical; have an irregular border; are uneven shades of brown, black, red, white, or blue; and are larger than six millimeters (about a quarter-inch) in diameter—can help you spot an abnormal mole while there is still time to do something about it. Reduce your risk by staying out of the sun, using a sunscreen, and covering up areas most susceptible to UV rays.

Hives

> **WHAT YOU SHOULD KNOW ABOUT...**
>
> ### Hives
> ➤ 20 percent of Americans will have an episode of hives.
> ➤ Hives are the body's reaction to a wide variety of foods, substances, and envi-ronments.
> ➤ Family history of hives places a person at higher risk.
> ➤ Red, raised welts are the distinguishing characteristics.
> ➤ Hives are treatable, temporary, and seldom life-threatening.

About one out of five people in the U.S. will have an episode of hives at some point. The American Academy of Dermatology explains that hives are produced by blood plasma leaking through very small gaps between the cells lining the small blood vessels in the skin. The condition manifests as red, raised areas on the skin in irregularly-shaped sizes ranging from very small to several inches across. These welts, which have a red border, can develop anywhere on the body, including the arms, legs, and trunk, either alone or in groups. Acute hives (urticaria is the scientific name) can last a few hours or a few weeks. When the condition lasts longer than six weeks, it is classified as chronic hives. In both cases, hives flare-ups come and go, only to appear somewhere else on the body.

A person most likely to suffer from hives has had a previous episode, tends to have allergic reactions in addition to those resulting in hives, has a family history of hives, or has a disorder such as lupus, lymphoma, or thyroid disease.

Acute hives

Acute hives are usually the body's reaction to certain foods (eggs, tomatoes, chocolate, nuts, milk, and shellfish, for example), medications (aspirin, penicillin, sulfa drugs, sedatives, antacids, laxatives, codeine, and others), stings (bees, wasps), or infections (hepatitis, strep throat, mononucleosis, colds). Physical factors such as heat, cold, sunlight, water, pressure on the skin, exercise, and emotional stress can also trigger episodes in 20 percent of cases.

Chronic hives

Not only do chronic hives last longer, but the cause is harder to detect. There is no specific test to identify the condition. In more than 80 percent of chronic cases, the cause is unknown, despite reviews of a patient's medical history, physical examinations, blood work, skin tests, and biopsies. In about half of those cases, the body's immune system triggers the release of histamines, which cause the fluid to leak from blood vessels and produce swelling.

In a related condition called angioedema, the swelling occurs underneath the skin rather than on top of it. Affected areas include the lips, eyes, hands, feet, and possibly the genitals. The swelling caused by angioedema sometimes may affect the throat, tongue, or lungs, and make breathing difficult. This life-threatening situation requires immediate medical attention.

Treatment

The good news about hives is that they are usually temporary and rarely life-threatening. The goal of treatment is to relieve the symptoms, and that may be done with cool compresses or showers, damp cloths, loose-fitting clothes, minimizing vigorous physical activity, and avoiding uncomfortably warm environments.

Over-the-counter (OTC) antihistamines like Benadryl, Chlor-Trimeton, Zyrtec, Tavist, and Claritin counter the effects of the histamine produced by the body, as can prescription drugs such as Atarax, Clarinex, Vistaril, Allegra, and Xyzal. These medications may be taken in combination with drugs known as histamine-2 (H2) blockers, such as Zantac and Tagamet. The corticosteroid prednisone, when taken orally, might control hives, but because of its side effects it is seldom recommended.

Before taking any OTC or prescription medications, let your doctor know which other drugs, including supplements, you are taking. Doing so could prevent drug interactions that could cause complications. Any type of drug therapy should be designed for your specific needs.

Prevention

Avoiding the substances and environments that cause hives is the best way to prevent them, but it's not always that easy. If you think foods are the problem, keep a diary to detect problem items or problem ingredients that they might contain.

Lupus

WHAT YOU SHOULD KNOW ABOUT...

Lupus

- Lupus affects 10 times as many women as men.
- A common symptom is a "butterfly" rash across the nose and cheeks.
- No single laboratory test can confirm the presence of lupus.
- Exposure to sunlight can trigger internal and skin responses.
- Most people with lupus live normal lives if they closely monitor their condi-tion and treat it to prevent complications.

Lupus is a chronic disease in which the body's immune system attacks its own healthy cells, tissues, and organs by mistake. There are four types of lupus, but the most common and serious form of the disease is systemic lupus erythematosus, which can affect many parts of the body, including the skin. Other potential targets are the joints, lungs, kidneys, and blood.

Lupus can affect anyone at any age, but women get it more often than men. It is diagnosed between ages 15 and 45 more than in other age groups, and it is more common in Asians and blacks than in other ethnic groups.

A skin rash is at the top of the list of symptoms, specifically one called a "butterfly rash," which is a reddish eruption across the bridge of the nose and cheeks. Other symptoms include fever, fatigue, and weight loss; a rash in an area exposed to sunlight; raised, scaly patches; arthritis involving multiple joints for several weeks; mouth or nose ulcers; kidney problems (detected with blood tests); anemia, low blood cell count, or low platelet counts; and seizures.

Because the symptoms vary from person to person, lupus is difficult to diagnose. Your family physician (or a rheumatologist) will compile a comprehensive medical history, conduct a physical exam, and put you through a battery of laboratory tests, but there is no single test that can absolutely confirm that a person has lupus.

Treatment

If and when lupus is diagnosed, treatment includes rest, exercise, physical therapy, and medications—NSAIDs, steroids, antimalarial drugs, and drugs that suppress the immune system. It is very important for a person who has lupus to avoid exposure to sunlight and UV rays emitted indoors by fluorescent and halogen lights.

Warts

Common warts, foot warts (also called plantar warts), and flat warts are all noncancerous growths caused by a viral infection. They can develop almost anywhere on the body and are usually the color of skin.

Common warts are more likely to appear on the hands, especially where the skin has been broken. Foot warts develop on the soles of the feet, but do not usually grow out of the skin because the pressure of walking pushes them back into the bottom surface of the foot. Flat warts are smooth and small, but as many as 100 can develop in a single area—often on the face in older men and on the legs of women. The warts may be associated with shaving those areas, but scientists have not been able to prove that theory.

Warts can be transmitted from one person to another, but the risk is very small. The time between contact with another person and developing a wart is several months. Contact doesn't have to be direct. Sharing towels and other items with a person who has warts could facilitate the transfer of the virus. Some warts go away on their own, while others have to be removed because they are causing a problem.

Treatment

Warts should be removed if they are unsightly, painful, or bleeding. One home remedy is to apply salicylic acid (contained in Compound W) to warts on the hands, feet, or knees, but the acid has to be applied every day for several weeks. Another folk remedy is covering a wart with duct tape to irritate the area and trick the body into attacking it. Duct tape is effective only about 20 percent of the time.

A doctor might apply a chemical called cantharidin to destroy the wart. A second visit is needed to remove the dead skin of the wart. Dermatologists also use liquid nitrogen to freeze a wart, and two to four treatments over a period of several weeks are necessary to completely remove the growth. Immunotherapy, laser therapy, and injecting each wart with an anti-cancer drug (bleomycin) are used less frequently than more conservative methods.

Sometimes, warts can reappear almost as fast as existing ones go away, probably because the virus is still present in the general area. The only way to deal with this problem is to treat the new growths as soon as possible to prevent the leftover virus from infecting nearby skin. If warts recur, see a dermatologist for professional help.

Other infections

Other skin infections include impetigo, folliculitis, herpes simplex, and scabies. People who sweat excessively (hyperhidrosis) are at a higher risk of fungal and bacterial infections, as well as atopic dermatitis.

Impetigo

Impetigo is caused by a bacterial infection that produces crusty skin lesions that itch first and ooze later. It is a common, contagious skin condition seen most often in children, but it can develop in adults who have had other skin disorders, colds, or upper respiratory infections. A doctor can usually diagnose impetigo simply by looking at it. Antibacterial creams are effective for mild infections, but more severe cases require oral antibiotics. The lesions seldom leave scars, even though they heal slowly. Prevent the spread of impetigo by using clean washcloths and towels and not sharing towels, clothing, razors, or anything else with friends or family members.

Folliculitis

When hair follicles are damaged by friction, blockage, or shaving, they can become infected with the staphylococcus (staph) bacteria. Symptoms include a rash, itching, or pimples on the neck, groin, or genital area. Your doctor may be able to diagnose folliculitis with a visual exam. Lab tests show the type of disease agent that has caused the infection. Hot, wet compresses can help drain the area, and treatment may include oral or topical antibiotics. The condition is easy to treat, but it may recur and the infection can spread to other areas of the body. If self-care doesn't relieve symptoms within two or three days, contact a medical professional.

Herpes simplex

The herpes simplex virus (HSV 1) causes cold sores and blisters around the mouth. (A different kind of herpes virus—herpes zoster—causes chickenpox and shingles, and herpes simplex type 2 causes genital herpes.) The sores may sting, burn, tingle, or itch. Many people become infected when they are exposed to the virus, but no more than 10 percent develop symptoms, which occur two to 20 days after contact with a person who has been infected. The blisters may heal on their own or they may break and allow fluid to drain. Creams and ointments usually work for mild cases. The scab, or crust, eventually falls off. The virus that caused the outbreak stays in the body and may reappear later. Prescription medications like acyclovir, famciclovir, and valacyclovir, taken orally, are effective for more serious cases. You can prevent HSV 1 by avoiding physical contact with an infected person and not sharing cups, glasses, or eating utensils with them.

Scabies

Older adults, especially those with weakened immune systems, are at a higher risk for scabies than younger, healthier people. Scabies is an infestation of the skin with a microscopic mite. It is a common condition found around the world and spreads rapidly in crowded conditions where there is frequent skin-to-skin contact. It could happen in hospitals, nursing homes, and other institutions, but prolonged contact is usually needed to transmit the infection. A casual handshake or hug is not likely to cause a problem. It could take four to six weeks after contact for symptoms to develop. The symptoms are skin irritation or a rash, usually between the fingers or on the wrists, elbows, knees, breasts, or shoulder blades. Your doctor can prescribe a topical cream or lotion that will get rid of the infestation, although the symptoms may last a week or two longer.

For more information

For more information about diagnosing, treating, and preventing skin conditions and diseases, see the list of organizations and their contact information that follows in Chapter 5. To subscribe to a free newsletter titled *Skin E-News*, published by the American Academy of Dermatology, go to www.aad.org/forms/NewsletterPublicSignUp/. ∎

5 GETTING HELP

You are the first line of defense against skin cancer or any other kind of skin condition, but not enough Americans are taking timely steps to protect themselves.

While 80 percent of adults are concerned about skin cancer and believe it is important to protect themselves, more than half (59 percent) have never been screened. Twenty-eight percent have never examined their own skin for changes to moles and other blemishes. One of the five risk factors leading to melanoma is the absence of regular visits to a dermatologist, and some people are simply too embarrassed to get a regular full-body skin cancer exam.

Of those who do get an exam, women are more likely to do so than men. Men over age 50 are in the highest risk group for melanoma, but often seek a screening only after having been previously diagnosed with skin cancer.

You can do at least three things to protect yourself. First, become more informed about potential problems. A glossary of terms appears in Appendix I, and a list of skin protection resources appears in Appendix II. Second, protect yourself by following the basic skin care guidelines described in Chapter 2. Third, conduct regular skin self-examinations.

The Skin Cancer Foundation (SCF) and the National Cancer Institute recommend monthly self-examinations and yearly exams performed by a dermatologist. Remember, the five-year cure rate for melanoma that has not spread to lymph nodes is 99 percent.

Self-exam instructions

To examine yourself, you'll need a bright light, full-length mirror, hand mirror, two chairs or stools, and a blow dryer. Here are instructions for conducting a self-exam provided by the SCF.

1. Examine your head and face, using one or both mirrors, and use the dryer to inspect your scalp.
2. Check your hands and nails, and use the full-length mirror to examine elbows, arms, and underarms.
3. Focus on your neck, chest, and torso. Women should check under their breasts.
4. With your back to a mirror, use the hand mirror to inspect the back of your neck, and your shoulders, upper arms, back, buttocks, and legs.
5. Sitting down and using the second chair or stool, check your legs, feet, soles, heels, and nails. Use the hand mirror to examine your genital area.

Having a partner assist in self-examinations makes it more likely that self-screening will occur and can improve the early detection of skin cancer. Men over 40 are not particularly accurate in spotting melanomas and may need help from a friend or spouse.

Seeing a doctor

The second line of defense is your family physician and/or a dermatologist. Your family doctor can answer general questions about skin health and potential skin problems, can treat minor skin problems such as rashes, and can refer you to a dermatologist when it is appropriate. Dermatologists can treat all of the skin conditions described in this report and should be seen for annual skin exams and for more serious skin conditions.

Scheduling an appointment with a dermatologist is not as easy as it sounds. The average patient will have to wait an average of 33 days to get an appointment. That number increases to 53 days to see a dermatologist at an academic clinic.

When examining skin biopsies and blood samples, dermatologists diagnose almost twice the number of skin lesions correctly (75 percent to 40 percent) as non-dermatologists. They correctly diagnose inflammatory skin diseases 71 percent of the time, compared to 34 percent for non-dermatologists. However, there is a shortage of dermatologists to meet the increasing demand of accurate melanoma screening.

The AAD encourages regular skin checkups for everyone, but says people who are at higher risk should be especially conscientious about getting medical help in evaluating skin conditions. Factors that place individuals in a high-risk group include:

- A family or personal history of skin cancer
- Exposure to ultraviolet (UV) rays over a period of time
- Severe sunburns
- Fair skin, blond or red hair, and blue, green, or gray eyes
- Sun-sensitive skin
- Large, irregularly shaped moles and/or 50 or more moles
- X-ray treatment for acne
- Taking drugs that suppress the immune system

A dermatologist is a doctor who specializes in treating conditions that affect the skin, hair, and nails. Many dermatologists have general practices and see patients with all types of skin concerns. Some dermatologists have had additional training in a specific area of dermatology, such as pediatrics, surgery, or cosmetics, and may have a practice that specializes in one of these areas.

What to take on the first visit

An increasing number of dermatologists allow patients to fill out forms online so that you don't have to balance that clipboard on your lap while sitting in the waiting room. Here is a checklist of documents you might be asked to present on your first visit:

- Photo ID
- Medical records from previous doctors (if they have not been forwarded directly to the dermatologist's office)
- List of prescription and over-the-counter medications you are taking
- List of vitamins, minerals, and other supplements you are taking
- X-rays, scans, and MRIs previously taken
- Lab test results
- List of prior surgeries and the dates on which they were performed
- List of questions to ask the doctor
- Insurance and/or Medicare card
- Checkbook or credit card to pay for the first visit

The doctor will ask questions about the nature of your skin condition, symptoms, how long it has existed, and what seems to make it worse. A Skin Condition Checklist allows you to record information in advance that might help your doctor evaluate your problem. Check each item that applies to your condition (see Box 5-1).

The exam

Dermatologists are trained to visually examine the skin, and may use a handheld dermoscope to get a closer look at moles or other suspicious growths. Your dermatologist also might photograph an area for use in later examinations to identify changes. When a lesion is suspected to be skin cancer, it will be removed and evaluated by a pathologist to confirm a diagnosis.

Organizations and institutions

In addition to local doctors, health care professionals, and health educators, use the Resources & Contact Information list in Appendix II to get more information about education, treatment, and prevention of skin cancer and other dermatological diseases. ■

BOX 5-1

Skin condition checklist

Place a check next to the words that apply to your condition:

Symptoms
- redness
- scales
- oily skin
- flaky skin
- itchy skin
- inflammation
- other

Location
- scalp
- eyebrows
- ears
- nose
- cheek
- back
- underarms
- groin, other

Duration
- days
- weeks
- months
- years

Severity
- slight
- mild
- moderate
- severe

Contributing factors
- stress
- fatigue
- illness
- travel
- weather changes
- medications
- foods/beverages
- other
- not sure

*Adapted with permission from Barrier Therapeutics

APPENDIX I: GLOSSARY

AAD: American Academy of Dermatology

actinic keratosis: a precancerous skin condition that is highly treatable when detected early

allergic contact dermatitis: a rash that appears when the body's immune system overreacts to foreign substances

alpha-hydroxy acids: acids derived from fruit and milk that are used in creams and lotions to try to reduce age spots, wrinkles, and other signs of aging

antioxidants: substances that protect cells from damage caused by free radicals, which are unstable molecules that could have a negative effect on skin health

atopic dermatitis: a skin disorder characterized by itching, scaling, and thickening of the skin that occurs in individuals predisposed to certain hypersensitivity reactions

basal cell carcinoma: the most common and most curable form of skin cancer

biochemotherapy: the use of immunotherapy in conjunction with chemotherapy

boil: a red, elevated, painful bump on the skin often caused by an infected hair follicle

callus: a condition caused by friction in which the skin has hardened or thickened, usually on toes, balls of the feet, heels, knees, or hands

chemotherapy: the use of drugs taken either orally or intravenously to kill cancer cells

collagen: fibers of protein found in connective tissue, cartilage, and bone

contact dermatitis: a rash caused by something a person has come in contact with, such as a chemical or poisonous plant

corn: a condition caused by friction, usually between the toes or on the top or outer sides of the toes

cosmeceutical: a product that has (or claims to have) both cosmetic and therapeutic benefits

cryotherapy: freezing an area of skin to destroy unwanted tissue, such as growths, moles, or warts

curettage-electrodesiccation: scraping off a cancerous area with a curette and burning any remaining cells with an electric current

dendritic cell: a type of special immune cell believed to be a major contributor to psoriasis

dermabrasion (surgical skin planing): a procedure used to wear away the layers of skin and improve irregularities on the surface of the skin

dermatologist: a physician who specializes in skin disorders

dermis: the middle layer of skin that contains nerves, blood vessels, oil glands, and hair follicles

dermoscope: a handheld microscope-like device that magnifies a pigmented lesion and allows the dermatologist to see through the outermost layer of skin

diabetic dermopathy: a skin disease specific to diabetes patients characterized by brown, scaly, oval or circular patches of skin on the front of the legs

elastin: a protein in the skin that helps maintain resilience and elasticity

epidermal cyst: a sac beneath the surface of the skin filled with keratin and fatty material

epidermis: the tough, outer protective layer of skin

eruptive xanthomatosis: a skin disease that occurs in severe cases of diabetes, characterized by small bumps on the skin surrounded by a red circle

excisional surgery: a procedure in which a lesion or growth is surgically removed

folliculitis: a damaged hair follicle infected with staphylococcus bacteria

herpes simplex: a virus that causes cold sores and blisters around the mouth

hives: an allergic reaction of the skin characterized by red, raised marks in irregular sizes ranging from very small to several inches

hyaluronic acid: a substance in connective tissues that cushions, lubricates, and provides volume to the skin

immunotherapy: treatment with medications that stimulate the immune system to fight skin cancer

impetigo: a skin infection caused by bacteria, characterized by skin lesions that itch first and ooze later

irritant contact dermatitis: a reaction that occurs when the skin is damaged by a foreign substance

laser therapy: the use of high-intensity light to treat several diseases, including basal cell skin cancer

Mohs micrographic surgery: a procedure in which skin is removed layer by layer and immediately examined for the presence of cancer cells

mole (nevus): a spot on the skin that contains melanin cells, which give color to the skin

necrobiosis lipoidica: a rare skin disease caused by a change in the blood vessels that affects people with diabetes

NSAIDs (nonsteroidal anti-inflammatory drugs): pain medications such as aspirin, ibuprofen or naproxen that relieve discomfort associated with sunburn and other painful skin conditions

photoaging: damage caused by sun exposure over a period of time

phototherapy: the use of natural or UV light to treat psoriasis and other conditions

psoriasis: a chronic, inflammatory, immune-related condition of the skin

psoriatic arthritis: a form of arthritis that occurs in 10 to 30 percent of people who have psoriasis

radiation therapy: the use of high-energy X-rays and other forms of radiation to kill cancer cells when the cancer has spread to other organs and tissue

rash: an area of irritated, red, scaly, crusty, blistered, or swollen skin caused by diseases, irritating substances, allergies, and your genetic makeup

retinoids: synthetic forms of vitamin A used to treat acne, aging skin, psoriasis, and certain skin cancers

rosacea: a skin condition characterized by red skin that resembles a sunburn

scabies: an infestation of the skin with a microscopic mite; more likely to affect older adults with weakened immune systems

seborrheic keratosis: a benign skin tumor that is very common in older adults

shingles: a disease caused by the herpes zoster virus, characterized by pain and a skin rash

skin tag: a benign, skin-colored growth on the skin; more common after age 60

squamous cell carcinoma: the second-most common form of skin cancer

subcutaneous layer (subcutis): the deepest layer of skin

sun protection factor (SPF): A measurement of a sunscreen's effectiveness equating to how many times longer a person wearing sunscreen can stay in the sun before beginning to burn than they can without any sunscreen at all

ultraviolet (UV) rays: radiation found in sunlight that can damage skin cells and cause sunburn, premature wrinkles, skin cancer, and other skin problems

ultraviolet protection factor (UPF): a measurement of how much ultraviolet radiation a particular clothing material absorbs

wart: a noncancerous growth on the skin caused by a viral infection

APPENDIX II: RESOURCES & CONTACT INFORMATION

Division of Dermatology David Geffen School of Medicine at UCLA
200 UCLA Medical Plaza
Suite 450
Los Angeles, CA 90095-6957
Phone: 310-917-3376

American Academy of Dermatology
P.O. Box 4014
Schaumburg, IL 60168-4014
Phone: 866-503-7546
www.aad.org

American Autoimmune Related Diseases Association, Inc.
22100 Gratiot Avenue
East Detroit, MI 48021
Phone: 586-776-3900
Phone: 800-598-4668
www.aarda.org

American Cancer Society
Phone: 800-227-2345
www.cancer.org

American Contact Dermatitis Society
2323 North State Street #30
Bunnell, FL 32110
Phone: 386-437-4405
www.contactderm.org
info@contactderm.org

American Skin Association
6 East 43rd Street, 28th Floor
New York, NY 10017
Phone: 212-889-4858
Phone: 800-499-SKIN
www.americanskin.org
info@americanskin.org

Basal Cell Carcinoma Nevus Syndrome Life Support Network (BCCNS)
P.O. Box 321
Burton, Ohio 44021
Phone: 866-834-1895
www.bccns.org
info@bccns.org

Centers for Disease Control and Prevention (CDC)
1600 Clifton Road
Atlanta, GA 30333
Phone: 404-639-3534
Phone: 1-800-311-3435
http://www.cdc.gov/ cdcinfo@cdc.gov

Lupus Foundation of America
2000 L Street, NW
Suite 710
Washington, DC 20036
Phone: 202-349-1155
Phone: 800-558-0121
www.lupus.org

Melanoma Research Foundation
1411 K Street, NW
Suite 500
Washington, DC 20005
Phone: 202-347-9675
Phone: 1-800-673-1290
www.melanoma.org
info@melanoma.org

Melanoma International Foundation
250 Mapleflower Road
Glenmoore, PA 19343
Phone: 866-463-6663
www.melanomaintl.org

National Cancer Institute NCI Public Inquiries Office
6116 Executive Boulevard
Suite 300
Bethesda, MD 20892-8322
Phone: 800-422-6237
www.cancer.gov
cancergovstaff@mail.nih.gov

National Institute on Aging
Building 31, Room 5C27
31 Center Drive, MSC 2292
Bethesda, MD 20892-8322
Phone: 301-496-1752
Phone: 800-222-2225
www.nia.nih.gov
nianews3@mail.nih.gov

National Institute of Arthritis and Musculoskeletal and Skin Diseases
1 AMS Circle
Bethesda, MD 20892-3675
Phone: 301-495-4484
Phone: 877-226-4267
www.niams.nih.gov
NIAMSInfo@mail.nih.gov

National Psoriasis Foundation
6600 SW 92nd Avenue
Suite 300
Portland, OR 97223-7195
Phone: 800-723-9166
www.psoriasis.org
getinfo@psoriasis.org

National Rosacea Society
196 James Street
Barrington, IL 60010
Phone: 888-NO-BLUSH
www.rosacea.org
lmartin@psoriasis.org

National Shingles Foundation
603 West 115 Street
Suite 371
New York, NY 10025
Phone: 212-222-3390
www.vzvfoundation.org
Shingles@ShinglesFoundation.org

Skin Cancer Foundation
149 Madison Avenue
Suite 901
New York, NY 10016
Phone: 212-725-5176
www.skincancer.org